☠ —A true emergency, as outlined above. Memorizing these conditions may help, rather than referring to this book when the patient is in the department! Call for immediate senior help. Try to remain calm and quickly assess the ABCs. Once the problem has been dealt with, remember to re-assess—other problems may have been forgotten or missed in the heat of the moment.

⚙ —These patients still need to be assessed very quickly, but you do not need to drop everything and run (so long as their ABCs have been managed). These patients can quickly shift into the emergency category if not sorted soon. Consider senior help/advice.

① —The majority of patients will fall into this and the last category. Although they do not need to be seen straight away, make sure you assess them thoroughly—some conditions can deteriorate if not treated properly. Think carefully of potential complications that may develop, such as atrioventricular block with inferior MIs or tamponade with pericardial effusions. Liaise with specialist help, if necessary.

② —These are non urgent conditions and general points of interest. Many of these patients, strictly speaking, should not come to casualty in the first place.

Emergencies in Obstetrics and Gynaecology

Edited by

S. Arulkumaran

Professor and Head of Obstetrics and Gynaecology,
St George's University of London, UK

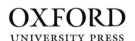

OXFORD

UNIVERSITY PRESS

OXFORD

UNIVERSITY PRESS

Great Clarendon Street, Oxford OX2 6DP

Oxford University Press is a department of the University of Oxford.
It furthers the University's objective of excellence in research, scholarship,
and education by publishing worldwide in

Oxford New York

Auckland Cape Town Dar es Salaam Hong Kong Karachi
Kuala Lumpur Madrid Melbourne Mexico City Nairobi
New Delhi Shanghai Taipei Toronto

With offices in

Argentina Austria Brazil Chile Czech Republic France Greece
Guatemala Hungary Italy Japan Poland Portugal Singapore
South Korea Switzerland Thailand Turkey Ukraine Vietnam

Oxford is a registered trade mark of Oxford University Press
in the UK and in certain other countries

Published in the United States
by Oxford University Press Inc., New York

British Library Cataloguing in Publication Data
Data available

Library of Congress Cataloging in Publication Data
Emergencies in obstetrics and gynaecology/edited by S. Arulkumaran.
    p. cm.—(Oxford medical publications)
Includes bibliographical references and index.
1. Obstetrical emergencies—Handbooks, manuals, etc. 2. Gynecologic
emergencies—Handbooks, manuals, etc. 3. Pregnancy—Complications—
Handbooks, manuals, etc.
  [DNLM: 1. Pregnancy Complications—Handbooks. 2. Emergencies—Handbooks.
3. Genital Diseases, Female—Handbooks. 4. Obstetrics—Handbooks. WQ 39 E53
2006] I. Arulkumaran, Sabaratnam. II. Series.
RG571.E462 2006
618.2'025–dc22   2006005946

Typeset by Newgen Imaging Systems (P) Ltd., Chennai, India
Printed in Italy
on acid-free paper by LegoPrint S.p.A.

ISBN 978–0–19–856730–1 (flexicover: alk paper)   0–19–856730–8 (flexicover: alk paper)

10 9 8 7 6 5 4 3 2 1

Preface

'Patient Safety' is one of the foremost agendas in many countries. About 3% to 10% of patients who enter hospitals for treatment end up with an unwanted, unexpected outcome as a result of medical accident. Such accidents are more common when emergencies are managed. Elective treatment provides the medical staff ample opportunity to reflect, consult, acquire further information, or refer for appropriate and better treatment. When faced with an emergency the best management has to be immediate. Adequate knowledge and skills are needed to deal with such emergencies.

This handbook provides the knowledge-base to manage emergencies in obstetrics and gynaecology. The topics covered may not be complete or comprehensive to deal with all emergencies, but are adequate for the common problems. There is deliberate overlap of general resuscitation measures within chapters and amongst other books in the same series. This is to emphasise its importance as a life-saving measure, and to provide a complete overview of management. Clinical problems that are of a semi-emergency nature that commonly present to out-patients clinics or GP surgeries are also covered. This, along with sections in pharmacotherapeutics in obstetrics and gynaecology should make this book a pocket companion to medical students and doctors working in obstetrics and gynaecology, general practice, and accident and emergency. The authors have written the chapters to suit the needs of the above and for those in the foundation years who have to acquire a broad knowledge-base on management of emergencies. The publishers and the editor would welcome constructive comments and criticism that will help to improve the next edition.

S. Arulkumaran

Acknowledgements

The editor would like to acknowledge the help of all the authors who have contributed to this book. Special thanks to Mrs Sue Cunningham of St. George's University of London who co-ordinated this project.

My sincere appreciation to Dr Séamus Sweeney, of St Patrick's Hospital, Dublin who reviewed the manuscripts and gave constructive comments. Special thanks to Catherine Barnes, Sara Chare, Helen Hill from OUP for their untiring efforts and patience in producing this book.

Contents

List of contributors

Rukma Bhattacharya
Specialist Registrar,
Torbay Hospital, Torquay, UK

Amarnath Bhide
Consultant Obstetrician and
Honorary Senior Lecturer,
St George's Hospital,
London, UK

Tom Bourne
Consultant Gynaecologist,
Early Pregnancy Unit,
St George's Hospital,
London, UK

Edwin Chandraharan
Honorary Senior Lecturer/
Consultant, St George's,
University of London, UK

James Clarke
Consultant Anaesthetist,
St George's Hospital, London, UK

George Condous
Clinical Fellow, Early Pregnancy Unit,
St George's Hospital, London, UK

Kate Farrer
Consultant Neonatologist,
St George's Hospital, London, UK

Michelle Fynes
Consultant Urogynaecologist,
St George's Hospital,
London, UK

Sarah Harper
Specialist Registrar,
Nottingham City Hospital,
Nottingham, UK

Kevin Hayes
Senior Lecturer and Honorary
Consultant in Obstetrics &
Gynaecology, St George's,
University of London, UK

Olujimi Jibodu
Consultant Obstetrician and
Gynaecologist, York Hospital,
York, UK

Emma Kirk
Clinical Fellow, Early Pregnancy
Unit, St George's Hospital,
London, UK

Krishna Kumar
Clinical Fellow in Maternal
Medicine, Espom and St Helier
Univeristy Hospitals NHS Trust,
Surrey, UK

Sandeep Mane
Consultant Obstetrician and
Gynaecologist, Convenor
of Basic Surgical Skills Course,
RCOG, London, UK

Edward Morris
Consultant Obstetrician &
Gynaecologist, Norfolk &
Norwich University Hospital,
Norwich , UK

Sambit Mukhopadhyay,
Consultant Obstetrician and
Gynaecologist, Norfolk & Norwich
University Hospital, Norwich, UK

Avidha Nejad
SpR in Obstetrics & Gynaecology,
Espom and St Helier University
Hospitals NHS Trust, Surrey, UK

Nicholas Ngeh
Specialist Registrar, Fetal Medicine
Unit, St George's Hospital,
London, UK

David Nunns
Consultant Gynaecological
Oncologist, Nottingham
City Hospital, Nottingham, UK

Penny Oakeley
Honorary Senior Lecturer in Family
Planning, St George's,
University of London, UK

Kamal Ojha
Consultant Obstetrician and
Honorary Senior Lecturer,
St George's Hospital, London, UK

Aris T. Papageorghiou
Lecturer in Obstetrics &
Gynaecology, St. George's,
University of London, UK

Leonie Penna
Consultant Obstetrician,
King's College Hospital, London, UK

Malini Prasad
Specialist Registrar in Obstetrics and
Gynaecology, Norfolk & Norwich
University Hospital, Norwich, UK

Hassan A. Shehata
Consultant and Honorary Senior
Lecturer in Maternal Medicine,
Epsom & St Helier University
Hospitals NHS Trust,
Surrey, UK

Jyothi Shenoy
Specialist Registrar in Obstetrics
and Gynaecology, The Queen
Elizabeth Hospital, King's
Lynn, UK

Abdul H. Sultan
Consultant Obstetrician and
Gynaecologist, Honorary Senior
Lecturer, Mayday University
Hospital, Croydon, UK

Onnig Tamizian
Consultant Obstetrician and
Gynaecologist, Derby City
General Hospital,
Derby, UK

Ranee Thakar
Consultant Obstetrician and
Urogynaecology Subspecialist,
Mayday University Hospital,
Croydon, UK

Austin Ugwumadu
Consultant Obstetrician
and Gynaecologist, St George's
Hospital, London, UK

Padma Vankayalapati
Clinical Fellow, Fetal
Medicine Unit, St George's
Hospital, London, UK

Barry Whitlow
Consultant Obstetrician &
Gynaecologist, Colchester
General Hospital,
Colchester, UK

Symbols and abbreviations

±	with/without
↑	increased
↓	decreased
°	degrees
>	greater than
<	less than
AC	abdominal circumference
ADH	antidiuretic hormone
AFI	amniotic fluid index
ALT	alanine aminotransferase
ARM	artificial rupture of membranes (amniotomy)
bds	2 times daily
BPD	bronchopulmonary dysplasia
BPP	biophysical profile
COCP	combined oral contraceptive pill
CRP	C-reactive protein
CTG	cardiotocograpgy
D&C	dilation and curettage
DCDA	dichorionic diamniotic twins
DIC	disseminated intravascular coagulation
DUB	dysfunctional uterine bleeding
ERPC	evacuation of retained products of conception
EUA	examination under anaesthetic
FBC	full blood count
FHR	fetal heart rate
FMH	fetomaternal haemorrhage
G&S	group and save
GA	general anaesthetic
GI	gastrointestinal
GIFT	gamete intrafallopian transfer
GTN	glycerol trinitrate
hCG	human chorionic gonadotrophin
HELLP	haemolysis, elevated liver enzymes, low platelet count
HIE	hypoxic ischaemic encephalopathy
ICSI	intracytoplasmic sperm injection
IHD	ischaemic heart disease
IUCD	intrauterine contraceptive device
IUD	intrauterine death

IUFD	intrauterine fetal death
IUGR	intrauterine growth restriction
IUS	intrauterine system
IVDA	intravenous drug abusers
IVF	in vitro fertilization
IVU	intravenous urogram
LFT	liver function test
LSCS	lower segment Caesarean section
MAS	movement alarm signal
MCDA	monochorionic diamniotic twins
MCMA	monochorionic monoamniotic twins
MI	myocardial infarction
MSU	mid-stream urine
NEC	necrotizing entercolitis
NST	non-stress test
od	once daily
PE	pulmonary embolism
PID	pelvic inflammatory disease
PP	placenta previa
PPH	postpartum haemorrhage
PPROM	pre-term, pre labour rupture of membranes
PROM	pre-labour rupture of the membranes
PSN	pre-sacral neurectomy
PVB	per vaginal bleeding
qds	4 times daily
RDS	respiratory distress syndrome
ROM	rupture of membranes
SABE	sub-acute bacterial endocarditis
SPD	symphysis pubis dysfunction
SROM	spontaneous rupture of membranes
STOP	suction termination of pregnancy
TCRE	transcervical resection of the endometrium
tds	3 times daily
TENS	transcutaneous electronic nerve stimulation
TOP	termination of pregnancy
TTTS	twin–twin transfusion syndrome
TVS	transvaginal scan
U	units
U&E	urea and electrolytes
UNA	uterine nerve ablation

☠ —A true emergency, as outlined above. Memorizing these conditions may help, rather than referring to this book when the patient is in the department! Call for immediate senior help. Try to remain calm and quickly assess the ABCs. Once the problem has been dealt with, remember to re-assess—other problems may have been forgotten or missed in the heat of the moment.

☼ —These patients still need to be assessed very quickly, but you do not need to drop everything and run (so long as their ABCs have been managed). These patients can quickly shift into the emergency category if not sorted soon. Consider senior help/advice.

① —The majority of patients will fall into this and the last category. Although they do not need to be seen straight away, make sure you assess them thoroughly—some conditions can deteriorate if not treated properly. Think carefully of potential complications that may develop, such as atrioventricular block with inferior MIs or tamponade with pericardial effusions. Liaise with specialist help, if necessary.

⑦ —These are non urgent conditions and general points of interest. Many of these patients, strictly speaking, should not come to casualty in the first place.

Obstetrics

Pregnancy changes and early pregnancy complications

⑦ Physiological changes in pregnancy

Pregnancy is a period of enormous physiological change in a relatively short space of time mediated by the endocrine (progesterone, oestrogens, cortisol, catecholamines, and HPL), paracrine (prostaglandins, cytokines), and physical effects of the utero-placental unit. They are well-tolerated by the majority of women. Understanding the normal changes can help to:

- Differentiate normality from the minority of women who experience pathological changes
- Explain the multitude of symptoms described in 'normal' pregnancy
- Explain the altered reference ranges in pregnancy for laboratory investigations and their subsequent interpretation
- Explain the different responses to some emergencies in pregnancy.

Cardiovascular changes

- Cardiac output increases by 40–50% (1500–2000 ml/min) by 10 weeks due to a large increase in stroke volume and a smaller increase in heart rate (overt tachycardia is not considered normal).
- There is a marked reduction in total peripheral resistance (systemic vasodilatation) resulting in reduced blood pressure (diastolic > systolic) in the first 2 trimesters returning to pre-pregnancy levels by the 3rd trimester.
- Venous pressure increases as uterine size increases (mass effect) explaining why up to 80% of women develop some leg oedema.

Haematological changes

- Plasma volume increases relatively more than red cell volume.
- Dilutional reduction in Hb concentration and haematocrit (maximal at 28–30 weeks).
- The term 'physiological anaemia of pregnancy' is erroneous.
- WHO definition of anaemia is Hb <10.5 g/dl and this requires investigation for underlying causes.
- Other changes in full blood count:
  - raised white count (neutrophilia)
  - 10–15% reduction in platelets
  - reduction in cell-mediated (lymphocytic) immunity and altered T:B cell ratio.
- Commonest cause of anaemia in pregnancy is iron deficiency (increased haematinic demand for iron around 4 mg/day unmasking underlying depletion or deficiency in iron stores).
- Iron absorption increases from 5–10% to 40% to meet demand (relies on adequate intake).
- Most women do not require iron supplementation.
- Folate deficiency unusual and B_{12} deficiency very rare (demand for both increased).
- Marked increases in coagulation factors VII, VIII, IX, X, XII, and particularly fibrinogen and a decrease in anti-thrombin III leading to a hypercoagulable state.

Respiratory changes
- Overall increase in ventilation (increased depth of ventilation more than respiratory rate). Mild respiratory alkalosis (CO_2 loss).
- Reduced diaphragmatic mobility in late pregnancy (especially in recumbent position).

Renal and urinary tract changes
- 40–50% increase in renal blood flow and glomerular filtration rate (by 1st trimester). Urea and creatinine concentrations are lower in normal pregnancy (larger excretion). Small reduction in serum sodium.
- Overall net gain in fluid balance (mineralocorticoid effect).
- Proximal tubular glucose reabsorption may be exceeded leading to glycosuria.
- Dilatation of ureters and pelvi-calyceal systems.

Gastrointestinal changes
- Gastro-oesophageal reflux is almost universal (reduced lower oesophageal tone).
- Gastric and intestinal motility reduced—'bloatedness' and constipation common.
- Liver function changes
  - increased placental alkaline phosphatase
  - reduction in serum albumin
  - reduction in ALT.

Metabolic changes
- E_2, HPL, and cortisol all induce insulin resistance.
- Hyperinsulinaemia leads to anabolism and storing of carbohydrate and fats.
- Susceptible individuals will develop glucose intolerance or frank gestational diabetes.

Clinical significance
- Large circulating volumes enable pregnant women to cope with hypovolaemia well and there may be minimal haemodynamic response to losses of up to 1000–1500 ml giving a false sense of security in the management of obstetric haemorrhage.
- Overall net fluid gains mean excessive use of oxytcin (ADH-like effect) can lead to fluid overload.
- The initial reduction in BP is less marked and the latter increase is exaggerated in pre-eclampsia due to poor initial vasodilatation and later vasoconstriction.
- The procoagulant state and pelvic mass effect are additive in increasing the risk of thromboembolic disease in pregnancy and the puerperium.
- Hb <10.5 g/dl needs investigation and antenatal correction to reduce risk at delivery from PPH.
- Some women describe tachypnoea and this may need to be differentiated from underlying causes such as cardio-respiratory disease or symptomatic anaemia.
- Repeated glycosuria is often physiological but may be an indicator of gestational diabetes.
- There is an overall degree of immunosuppression predisposing to sepsis.

☠ Pain/bleeding in early pregnancy

All women who present with lower abdominal pain and/or bleeding per vagina (PVB) in the reproductive age group must have a pregnancy test. If pregnant and in their 1st trimester, ideally they must have a transvaginal scan (TVS). This confirms viability, gestation, and, most importantly, the location of the pregnancy.

Ectopic pregnancy

- A diagnosis of ectopic pregnancy should be considered in any woman of reproductive age presenting with abdominal pain ± PVB who has a positive pregnancy test.
- Incidence is 9.6/1000 pregnancies in the United Kingdom (UK). Mortality is 4/1000 ectopic pregnancies and is responsible for over 75% of 1st trimester pregnancy deaths.[1] Over 10 000 ectopic pregnancies are diagnosed annually in the UK.
- Although collapse of a woman in the reproductive age group is uncommon, this should be considered to be due to an ectopic pregnancy until proven otherwise.

Risk factors

- Previous ectopic pregnancy
- History of pelvic inflammatory disease, chlamydia, or gonorrhoea
- History of infertility
- Previous tubal surgery (including tubal ligation)
- Assisted conception (e.g. IVF, GIFT, ICSI)
- Intra-uterine contraceptive device in situ
- The use of emergency contraception in this pregnancy.

Symptoms and signs

The following 'classical triad of symptoms' may be present:
- Amenorrhoea
- Lower abdominal pain (unilateral or bilateral)
- PVB.

However, most women with an ectopic pregnancy in modern practice are clinically stable at presentation and have non-specific symptoms. Other symptoms may include shoulder tip pain, which is a reflection of significant haemoperitoneum with blood irritating the diaphragm.

- Abdominal palpation may be unremarkable or, less commonly, confirm an acute abdomen with rebound tenderness, and in some cases guarding.
- Vaginal examination may be unremarkable or, less commonly, confirm cervical excitation, adnexal tenderness, or, very rarely, an adnexal mass.

Investigations

- Qualitative urinary hCG is almost always positive in an ectopic prenancy.
- Quantitative serum hCG is useful if urinary test is equivocal. It is important to quantify hCG levels in order to decide management strategy or confirm successful resolution of trophoblastic tissue after treatment.
- Serum progesterone <20 nmol/L indicates a probable failing pregnancy.
- FBC, G&S—transfusion may be required, rhesus negative women should receive anti-D immunoglobulin 250 IU.
- TVS is the diagnostic tool of choice.

Management

Depends on the clinical state of the woman. If a woman is haemodynami-cally compromised, resuscitation (Airway, Breathing, Circulation) is essential with concurrent transfer to the operating theatre for emergency surgery (usually a laparotomy). If a woman is stable, a TVS should be performed and this will confirm the diagnosis in more than 90% of women with an ectopic pregnancy. This is based upon the positive visualization of an adnexal mass, rather than the absence of an intra-uterine sac.

The combination of TVS with quantitative serum hCG levels are well-described diagnostic tools. Laparoscopy should be used to confirm TVS findings and treat tubal ectopic pregnancies rather than as a diagnostic tool.

TVS should not be performed in a clinically unstable woman, thus delaying theatre.

1. **Surgical treatment**
   - Indications: haemodynamic instability, pain, a viable ectopic pregnancy on TVS, haemoperitoneum on TVS, hCG >5000 U/L.
   - Laparoscopy preferable to laparotomy—decreased admission time, shorter post-operative recovery, and reduced analgesic requirements.
   - Whether salpingectomy or linear salpingotomy should be performed is uncertain. Recent studies show a higher subsequent intrauterine pregnancy rate with linear salpingotomy.

2. **Medical treatment (methotrexate) in selected patients**
   - Indications: asymptomatic, hCG <5000 U/L, no fetal cardiac activity on TVS, no haemoperitoneum on TVS, non-tubal ectopic pregnancies.
   - Most commonly given as a single intramuscular dose of 50 mg/m^2 of body surface area. Treatment successful if hCG decreased >15% between days 4–7 post injection. Success rates are between 65–95%.[2] May also be given intra-amniotically under TVS guidance or locally at the time of laparoscopy but this has no advantage over a systemic approach.

3. **Expectant treatment—'Wait and see' approach in selected patients**
   - Indications: asymptomatic, hCG <5000 U/L, decreasing hCG level, no fetal cardiac activity on TVS.
   - Successful in 48–70% cases, especially if hCG <175 U/L and progesterone <10nmol/L.[2,3]

Other causes of pain in early pregnancy

Ovarian cyst—haemorrhagic, rupture, bleeding, or torsion

Tender discrete mass in lower abdomen or adnexal mass on vaginal examination. Need TVS and pregnancy test to distinguish from ectopic pregnancy. The vast majority of ovarian cysts in the 1st trimester are physiological and resolve spontaneously.

Urinary tract Infection

Dysuria, increased frequency, urgency of micturition and suprapubic pain.

Appendicitis

Low grade pyrexia, nausea/vomiting, anorexia, paralytic ileus, pain worse on right side, rebound tenderness, guarding.

Miscarriage

Bleeding in the 1st trimester affects over 20–30% of pregnancies. Up to 50% of those who bleed will go on to have a miscarriage. 10–15% of clinically recognised pregnancies will miscarry.

Causes

- In the majority there is no demonstrable cause.
- Known causes include: chromosomal abnormality, abnormal placental development, multiple pregnancy, uterine abnormality, corpus luteum failure, infection.

Symptoms and signs

- PVB—may only be spotting or can be heavy with clots.
- Pain or cramping in lower abdomen, possibly radiating to back.
- Weakness, dizziness, collapse—vasovagal attacks may occur if products of conception are in the cervical os.

Investigations

- Physical examination—including speculum and bimanual pelvic examination. The uterus may be smaller than expected for dates. The cervical os may be open or closed. There may be products of conception within the cervical os that need removal.
- TVS is essential for ultrasound clssification of miscarriage—may demonstrate a sac with or without a fetal pole, retained products of conception or an empty uterus.
- Serial serum hCG—needed if no evidence of an intra-uterine pregnancy seen on TVS in order to exclude an ectopic pregnancy.
- Full blood count and sample for group and save.

Clinical classification of miscarriage is misleading and not helpful. A threatened miscarriage is a clinical diagnosis and always requires ultrasound follow-up. Classification should therefore be ultrasound-based as this confirms a diagnosis:

1. *Viable intra-uterine pregnancy*—fetal pole with cardiac activity
2. *Early intra-uterine pregnancy*—gestational sac with mean diameter <20 mm or fetal pole <6 mm without cardiac activity—rescan > 10 days to confirm viability
3. *Incomplete miscarriage*—heterogeneous tissue within the uterine cavity
4. *Anembryonic pregnancy or blighted ovum* (early embryonic demise)—empty gestational sac with mean diameter >20 mm
5. *Missed miscarriage* (early fetal demise)—fetal pole >6 mm with no cardiac activity
6. *Pregnancy of unknown location*—empty uterus—needs serial hCG to confirm whether complete miscarriage, an early pregnancy too early to visualize, or ectopic pregnancy.

Management

Depends on the clinical state of the woman and the presenting symptoms and signs. As with an ectopic pregnancy, resuscitation in an emergency situation may be necessary. Immediate removal of products from the cervical os for pain relief and vagal response may be helpful.

1. **Surgical (evacuation of retained products of conception—ERPC)**
   May be performed as an elective day case procedure or as an emergency if needed.

2. **Expectant**
   Highest success rates are in women with incomplete miscarriages. Majority of women in this group will complete their miscarriage within 2 weeks. Women with a missed miscarriage or an anembryonic pregnancy have only a 50% chance of resolving their pregnancy within 2 weeks.[4,5]

3. **Medical**
   Usually in the form of prostaglandin analogues (misoprostol or gemeprost), with or without antiprogesterone priming (mifepristone). Success rates vary from 13–96%[5]. Again success depends on type of miscarriage, with highest success rates in incomplete miscarriage.

4. **Anti-D immunoglobulin**
   Needed in Rhesus negative women over 12 weeks with any bleeding and in any women having surgical intervention.

5. **Psychological**
   Pregnancy loss can be an extremely distressing time for both the woman and her partner so it is important that there are resources available to offer counseling and support as necessary.

Other causes of bleeding in early pregnancy

Ectopic pregnancy
See above.

Pregnancy of unknown location
Defined with TVS as there being no signs of either an intra- or extra-uterine pregnancy or retained products of conception in a woman with a positive urinary pregnancy test. Management is expectant and based upon serum measurements of hCG and progesterone.

Molar pregnancy (gestational trophoblastic disease)
Most often diagnosed following histological assessment of products of conception and should be referred to tertiary trophoblastic unit (Charing Cross, Sheffield, or Dundee).

Cervical pathology
Cervical polyps, ectropion, infective cervicitis, carcinoma.

Infection
Vaginal candidiasis, chlamydia.

Implantation bleeding
Small amount of bleeding associated with the normal implantation of the embryo. Frequently on day period would have been due.

References

1. Confidential Enquiry into Maternal and Child Health (2004). Why Mothers Die 2000–2002: The Sixth Report of the Confidential Enquiry into Maternal Death in the United Kingdom. RCOG Press, London.
2. Kirk E et al. The non-surgical management of ectopic pregnancy. Ultrasound Obstet Gynecol 2006; **27**: 91–100.
3. Elson J et al. (2004). Expectant management of tubal ectopic pregnancy: prediction of successful outcome using decision tree analysis. Ultrasound Obstet Gynecol, 23, 552–6.
4. Luise C et al. (2002). Outcome of expectant management of spontaneous first trimester miscarriage: observational study. BMJ, **324**, 873–5.
5. Condous G et al. (2003). The conservative management of early pregnancy complications: a review of the literature. Ultrasound Obstet Gynecol, **22**, 420–30.

:✪: Vomiting in pregnancy

Nausea and vomiting in pregnancy are common early symptoms of pregnancy and are believed to be due to physiological hormonal changes of the pregnant state.

However, excessive vomiting may result in dehydration and electrolyte and metabolic derangements that can compromise maternal and fetal well-being. Many medical and surgical emergencies may present with vomiting during pregnancy and thus pose a diagnostic difficulty. It is essential to identify the underlying cause early so that appropriate treatment can be instituted.

Causes

Physiological

Emesis gravidarum: this refers to the nausea and vomiting of pregnancy that normally occurs around 8–10 weeks, with the peak of serum hCG levels. There is no electrolyte or metabolic derangements and the condition often settles by 12 weeks.

Pathological

Any vomiting that is excessive or continuing beyond 20 weeks should be considered pathological unless proven otherwise.

- Hyperemesis gravidarum: refers to any nausea and vomiting of pregnancy that is severe enough to cause dehydration, electrolyte and metabolic derangements that may endanger the life of the patient. This normally occurs around 8–10 weeks, may continue beyond 12 weeks, but rarely after 20 weeks. Multiple pregnancy and gestational trophoblastic disease (hydatidiform mole, choriocarcinoma) need to be excluded.
- Obstetric: severe pre-eclampsia/obstetric cholestasis/acute polyhydramnios.
- Gynaecological: torsion of ovarian cyst/pedunculated fibroid. Acute red degeneration of fibroid.
- Infections: urinary tract infections (pyelonephritis), chorioamnionitis, hepatitis, acute pancreatitis, gastrointestinal (including acute appendicitis), CNS infections (meningitis, encephalitis, cerebral malaria—in developing countries), viral infections.
- Metabolic: diabetic ketoacidosis, hyperthyroidism.
- Others: CNS tumours (pituitary adenoma), GI tumours (e.g. gastric cancer), intestinal obstruction, gastro-oesophageal reflux.

Psychological

Attention seeking /lack of family support.

History

? Known metabolic disorders, assisted reproduction.

Type of vomiting: ?projectile (raised intracranial pressure).

Associated factors:
- Nausea: GI disorders, malignancies, metabolic disorders.
- Dyspepsia: acute gastritis/gastric ulcer.
- Fever: infections/red degenration of fibroid.
- Pain: infections/torsion/red degeneration/polyhydramnios.
- Dysuria/pyuria/haematuria/loin to groin pain: UTI.
- Jaundice/loss of appetite: hepatitis/cholestasis.
- Headaches/visual disturbances: CNS tumours/pre-eclampsia.
- Tremors/sweating/anxiety: hyperthyroidism.
- Confusion/delirium/acetone breath: diabetic ketoacidosis.
- Constitutional symptoms: viral infections.
- Haematemesis: gastro-oesophageal reflux, gastric cancer, lower oesophageal tears due to excessive vomiting (Malory–Weiss Syndrome).

Examination
General condition
- Level of consciousness (?delirious/comatose, abnormal behaviour)
- Deep breathing (Kussmaul's breathing) ?acetone breadth
- Level of hydration
- ?icterus/?in pain.

Vital signs
pulse/BP/temperature/respiration.

Systemic examination
CVS/RS/CNS if pathology is suspected.

Abdominal examination
- Abdominal distension (if more than the uterine distension—?fluid or flatus due to intestinal obstruction).
- Guarding/rebound tenderness (peritonitis).
- Tenderness: suprapubic/renal angle/epigastric/right hypochondrial/uterine/iliac fossae/McBurney's point.
- Abdominal masses (e.g. lump in epigastric region with gastric cancer).
- Fluid thrill.

Investigations
- Urine dipstick—to exclude UTI, ketonuria
- Exclude infections—FBC, C-reative protein (CRP)
- Severity of vomiting—blood urea and serum electrolytes, serum creatinine, packed cell volume (haematocrit)
- Ultrasound scan—to exclude multiple pregnancy, gestational trophoblastic disease or adnexal masses.

Additional investigations—depending on the suspected aetiology
- Midstream sample of urine for microscopy & culture *(UTI)*
- Blood gases *(diabetic ketoacidosis)*
- Thyroid function tests *(hyperthyroidism)*
- Fasting/random blood glucose *(diabetic ketoacidosis)*
- Serum amylase *(pancreatitis)*
- Liver function tests *(hepatitis, severe pre-eclampsia, cholestasis)*

- Hepatitis serology *(hepatitis)*
- Abdominal ultrasound *(pyelonephritis, hepatitis, cholestasis)*
- Blood cultures *(chorioamnionitis, pyelonephritis)*
- Blood for malarial parasites *(malaria endemic areas)*
- Visual field testing/MRI scan *(CNS tumours)*
- Lumbar puncture *(CNS infection)*.

Sequelae
- Maternal and fetal compromise due to electrolyte and metabolic derangements.
- Metabolic acidosis with multi-organ failure.
- Wernicke's Encephalopathy and Korsakoff's Psychosis due to severe intractable vomiting.
- Maternal collapse and death in severe cases, if untreated.

Management
All patients with severe or intractable vomiting and/or with ketonuria need to be admitted. The principles of management of severe vomiting in pregnancy are given below:
- immediate correction of dehydration (hypovolumia), electrolyte and metabolic derangements.
- medications to stop further vomiting.
- specific management of the aetiology—may require a 'multi-disciplinary' approach.
- counselling and improving the psychological well-being.

Immediate correction of dehydration (hypovolumia), electrolyte and metabolic derangements
- Rapid intravenous infusion of 1L of normal saline or 5% dextrose solution.
- Addition of 20–40 mmol/L of potassium based on the serum electrolyte result.
- Continuation of intravenous fluids until there is a clinical improvements in the degree of dehydration, disappearance of ketones in the urine, decrease in the haematocrit, and when the patient is able to tolerate oral fluids.
- If diabetic ketoacidosis is confirmed, insulin needs to be administered via a separate infusion pump (with potassium), usually at a rate of 1 unit/hour—in conjunction with a diabetic physician. A sliding scale is mandatory. Patient may need sodium bicarbonate infusion to neutralize the metabolic acidosis.

Medications to stop further vomiting
- Metoclopamide 10 mg (iv/im/oral) 8 hourly—patient needs to be counselled regarding extra-pyramidal side effects.
- Cyclizine 50 mg (iv/im/oral) 8 hourly.
- Domperidone 10 mg (oral) 8 hourly or 60 mg bd (PR).
- Pyridoxine (vitamin B1) 10 mg—may help to reduce severe nausea.
- Antacids (ranitidine 50 mg IV/IM or cimetidine 200 mg IV/IM) may help reduce acute gastritis secondary to severe vomiting or if peptic ulcer disease is suspected.

- Thiamine 50 mg to prevent the development of Wernicke's encephalopathy and Korsakoff's psychosis, which are the dreaded complications of severe vomiting in pregnancy.

In intractable vomiting the following drugs may be administered
- Ondansetron 4 mg (IV/oral)—not licenced in pregnancy.
- Methyl prednisolone.

Specific management of the aetiology—may require a 'multi-disciplinary' approach

- Antibiotics—for UTI, chorioamnionitis.
- Evacuation of the hydatidiform mole when the condition is stable.
- Bromocriptine/cabergoline (pituitary adenoma) or surgery for CNS tumours.
- Medical management of hepatitis, pancreatitis, degenerating fibroid, cerebral malaria.
- Surgical management of acute appendicitis, intestinal obstruction and torsion of ovarian cysts or pedunculated fibroids.

Conclusion

Vomiting in pregnancy is a common disorder and is often due to physiological (hormonal) changes of pregnancy. However, it is important to be aware of the pathological causes of vomiting in pregnancy, some of which are medical or surgical emergencies. Clinical suspicion, early diagnosis, and appropriate emergency management may avoid unnecessary morbidity and mortality.

Medical emergencies in pregnancy

James Clarke

Aris T. Papageorghiou and S. Arulkumaran

Hassan Shehata and Krishna Kumar

Onnig Tamizian

Jyothi Shenoy and Sambit Mukhopadhyay

☠ **ABC of resuscitation in pregnancy**

- Cardiac arrest occurs in about 1:30 000 pregnancies.
- The survival of the mother and fetus depends on the management in the first critical minutes.
- All obstetricians should be able to diagnose cardiac arrest and start basic CPR.
- All obstetricians should be able to recognize *impending* cardio-respiratory arrest and institute appropriate measures to prevent deterioration into an arrest.

ABC of Resuscitation (Basic Life Support)[1]

A. Airway.   Is the airway clear?
B. Breathing.   Is chest moving or air movement at lips?
C. Circulation. Can you feel a carotid or femoral pulse?

If there is no circulation
- Start CPR resuscitation immediately
- Call cardiac arrest team
- For pregnant women > than 24 weeks there are 2 further important actions that must be undertaken:

D. Displacement of the gravid uterus to decrease effect of aortocaval compression on venous return
E. Emergency Caesarean section within 5–10 min of arrest if initial resuscitation is unsuccessful.

Airway
- Clear airway of debris/dentures/vomit.
- Tilt head back and thrust lower jaw forward, moving base of tongue from posterior pharyngeal wall creating clear passage from lips to larynx.

Breathing
If patient is breathing—place in coma position.
If patient is **not** breathing commence artificial ventilation immediately.
- Mouth-to-mouth
- Mouth-to-nose
- Face-mask and self-inflating bag (100% oxygen)
- Laryngeal mask with self-inflating bag (100% oxygen)
- Once expert help is available the patient's trachea should be intubated as soon as possible to prevent possible aspiration of gastric contents.
Ventilation should be at a rate of 2 breaths to 15 chest compressions.

Circulation

- To be effective, cardiac massage must be carried out on a firm surface. If necessary place patient on the floor.
- Cardiac massage is more difficult in the pregnant patient because of displacement of the diaphragm and rib cage by the gravid uterus.
- Compression should be carried out mid sternum to avoid possible damage to the liver[2].

Chest compression should be carried out at a rate of 100/min.

Changes in maternal physiology that may adversely affect resuscitation

- Maternal oxygen demands in the latter half of pregnancy are 20% higher than in the non-pregnant state.
- Cardiac output is 40% higher than non-pregnant state.
- The gravid uterus makes ventilation more difficult.
- 10% of maternal cardiac output goes to uterus and fetus.
- Ineffective resuscitation may result in a hypoxic fetus.

Displacement of gravid uterus[2]

With the patient lying on her back, aortocaval compression by the gravid uterus will decrease venous return, making effective resuscitation difficult. To decrease aortocaval compression without compromising effective cardiac massage employ one of the following methods.

- Manual displacement of the uterus anteriorly
- Use of a Cardiff wedge
- Place a folded pillow under the right buttock
- Place inverted chair under right buttock
- Whilst kneeling insert knees under right buttock
- Emergency CS.

Emergency Caesarean section

If resuscitation has not produced a spontaneous cardiac output within 5 minutes, an emergency Caesarean section should be carried out in situ. Full resuscitation should continue during the Caesarean section. This has the advantages of—

- Probably saving the baby's life (see table) if performed in less than 10 minutes
- Decreasing aortocaval compression thus increasing chances of successful maternal resuscitation
- Improving chest wall compliance, thus improving maternal oxygenation.

Fetal outcome following perimortem Caesarean Sections. Adapted from Katz et al. (1986)[3]

Time from arrest (min)	Number of patients	Outcome
0–5	42	Normal infants
6–10	7	Normal infants
	1	Mild neurological damage
11–15	6	Normal infants
	1	Severe neurological damage
16–20	1	Severe neurological damage
21+	2	Severe neurological damage

Cardiopulmonary bypass

- There are a number of case reports of successful resuscitation using cardiopulmonary bypass in obstetric patients.
- If available it should be considered.
- Is the method of choice in local anesthetic toxicity, as drug is bound to myocardium for up to 2 hours, making resuscitation prolonged and difficult.

Training

- There is some evidence that regular drills in cardiac arrest management in pregnancy can improve clinicians' confidence and possibly outcome.

References

1. Standards for Clinical Practice and Training (2004). Resuscitation Council (UK), London. www.resus.org.uk
2. Morris S, Stacey M (2003). Resuscitation in pregnancy. *BMJ*, **327**, 1277–9.
3. Katz VL, Dotters DJ, Droegemueller W (1986). Perimortem Cesarean delivery. *Obstet Gynecol*, **68**, 571–6.

Adult basic life support algorithm

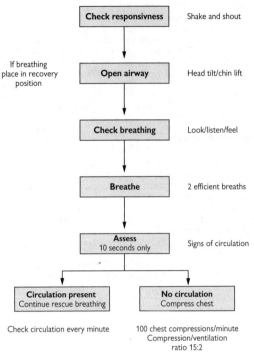

Reproduced with kind permission of the Resuscitation Council (UK)[1]

⊕ Abdominal pain in pregnancy

Abdominal pain is a common complaint during pregnancy. Labour itself is a common cause and it is usually intermittent in nature with associated uterine contractions. The definition of labour is regular uterine contractions with cervical effacement or dilatation, and descent of the presenting part. However, cervical change may be preceded by a long latent phase of labour, and this may make the diagnosis more difficult. The fact that abdominal pain is common and often physiological in pregnancy can mean that pathological causes are often overlooked. Remember that pathological conditions can co-exist with and even precipitate labour.

The causes can be divided into those caused by pregnancy, and those that are incidental to pregnancy.

Pregnancy-related causes
Physiological
- Labour: painful regular uterine contractions should be accompanied by cervical effacement or dilatation, and descent of the presenting part.
- Musculoskeletal pain from ligament stretching: this affects as many as 30% of pregnancies, and is more common in early and late gestation. It is usually stabbing in nature and aggravated by movement.
- Constipation: this is a common condition, affecting up to a third of all pregnancies at some gestation. It is thought to be due to hormonal changes in pregnancy causing decreased bowel motility and increased absorption of water. Iron supplements can often worsen symptoms. The patient's history is usually sufficient to make the diagnosis, and there is frequently a history of pre-existing constipation. Conservative treatment and dietary advice usually improves the condition, but bulking agents and in some cases stool softeners or stimulant laxatives may become necessary.

Pathological
- Ectopic pregnancy (see pp. 6–7)
- Miscarriage (see pp. 8–9)
- Placental abruption (see pp. 64–65)
- Chorioamnionitis.
- This may be accompanied by maternal pyrexia and tachycardia, leukocytosis or elevation of C-reactive protein, and fetal tachycardia. A history of prelabour rupture of the membranes (PROM) should raise the index of suspicion, but chorioamnionitis can also occur with no history of PROM. If there is evidence of chorioamnionitis, treatment with antibiotics should not delay the decision for delivery of the fetus regardless of gestational age, as the maternal condition can deteriorate rapidly.
- Complications of uterine fibroids: pain due to red degeneration or torsion of fibroids is usually localized, but can be very severe and may mimic placental abruption. Conservative management with analgesia (often opiates are required) and bedrest will usually allow spontaneous resolution of the symptoms. Laparotomy for both diagnosis and treatment is rarely required.

- Symphysis pubis dysfunction (SPD): this common condition of unknown aetiology usually causes pain and tenderness over the symphysis pubis joint. Pain may radiate to the hips, groin, lower abdomen, and lower back. Walking and weight-bearing on one leg (for example climbing stairs, getting in and out of bed) are particularly painful. Apart from analgesia, the mainstay of treatment is specialist physiotherapy that can provide support belts, transcutaneous electronic nerve stimulation (TENS), and crutches to aid mobility.

- Uterine rupture or scar dehiscence: this is an uncommon cause of pain, and can be difficult to diagnose as it is usually (but not always!) associated with labour. In most instances the pain occurs in the 3rd trimester, and there is a history of previous Caesarean section. However, rupture of the uterus can occur in women without previous Caesarean, and this is associated with multiparity, induction agents (prostaglandins and oxytocics), obstructed labour, or other previous uterine surgery, e.g. myomectomy. There is constant pain and scar tenderness even between uterine contractions, and this is often associated with vaginal bleeding that can be severe and can rapidly lead to maternal shock. Classically there is loss of the presenting part on vaginal examination. Abnormalities in the CTG are often the first clue to impending rupture or ruptured uterus. The treatment is by aggressive resuscitation, prompt laparotomy and delivery, and subsequent repair of the uterine defect. Rarely hysterectomy may be necessary.

  The condition can present, albeit rarely, in the immediate postnatal period. This will usually be with with signs of vaginal or intra-abdominal bleeding and shock. Delay in performing laparotomy can have catastrophic consequences.

- Uterine torsion: this is a rare cause of pain, and is caused either by rapid rotation of the uterus, or by rotation of over 90°. This will often be due to an associated uterine abnormality, uterine fibroids, or a large adnexal mass. Symptoms include abdominal pain, and a tender and firm uterus. Associated abnormalities in the CTG are often present, and this can make the condition difficult to distinguish from placental abruption. Clues are a more gradual onset of pain, urinary retention, and a lateral displacement of the urethra on catheterization. In severe cases Caesarean section may be necessary, but at earlier gestation expectant management with analgesia and altering of maternal position can be successful in prolonging pregnancy.

- Pre-eclampsia: one of the symptoms of pre-eclampsia is epigastric pain, which is due to stretching of the liver capsule. The presence of this symptom in severe pre-eclampsia or HELLP syndrome is an ominous sign and must be taken seriously, as it increases the risk of subcapsular hepatic bleeding or liver rupture.

- Acute fatty liver of pregnancy: this is a rare cause of acute severe liver disease of unknown cause, occurring in about 1 in 10 000 pregnancies. It usually presents in the late 3rd trimester, with epigastric or right upper quadrant abdominal pain, jaundice, nausea, and vomiting. Tiredness and confusion are often present, and can be signs of hepatic encephalopathy. Abnormal liver function or clotting may need to be followed by ultrasound of the liver for diagnosis. There are risks of maternal liver failure and coagulopathy, and fetal demise. Seek advice from a specialist liver unit early. Timely delivery will allow intensive care for the mother. In most cases the condition improves with supportive measures and liver function returns to normal within a few weeks. Rarely liver failure may ensue and transplantation becomes necessary. (Also see p. 47–48.)

Causes unrelated to pregnancy

Gastrointestinal tract

- Appendicitis: a common cause of an acute abdomen. It affects about 1 in 1000 pregnancies. It can be a challenging diagnosis because:
  - the position of the appendix changes in pregnancy and is behind the broad ligament obscuring guarding and rebound tenderness.
  - commonly there is absence of localization of pain.
  - nausea and vomiting are common in pregnancy as it is with appendicitis.
  - there is physiological leucocytosis in pregnancy.

  Absence of leukocytosis may be reassuring. Pyrexia, nausea, vomiting, tachycardia, coated tongue, and right-sided abdominal pain should raise the index of suspicion. Tenderness over the caecal area on per rectal examination suggests peritoneal inflammation. Delay in diagnosis can cause appendix rupture with resultant peritonitis (maternal mortality >10%) and premature labour or miscarriage. The risks of delayed diagnosis must be carefully balanced against the risks of surgical intervention on the mother and fetus. Ultrasound can be useful to exclude other causes, and can be suggestive of appendicitis, especially in the 1st trimester. Early surgical referral is essential.
- Acute cholecystitis: it is not uncommon and occurs in around 1 in 1500 pregnancies. Symptoms include right upper quadrant or epigastric pain with nausea, vomiting, and fever. Clinical jaundice is uncommon, but bilirubin and transaminases are usually elevated. The presence of cholelithiasis in most cases helps to differentiate it from obstetric cholestasis, acute fatty liver, and HELLP syndrome. Conservative management using antibiotics and analgesia is adequate in most cases. In more severe cases cholecystectomy, which can be done using open laparoscopy in the 1st and early 2nd trimester, may become necessary. (Also see p. 53–54.)
- Acute pancreatitis: this is rare in pregnancy (1 in 3000) and almost always occurs in the 3rd trimester. Classical symptoms include epigastric pain radiating to the flanks, shoulders, or back. Serum amylase can be elevated in pregnancy, but a very high level will confirm the diagnosis. Most cases will resolve within a few days with conservative treatment: intravenous fluids, analgesia, antibiotics, nasogastric suction, and nil orally.
- Intestinal obstruction: uncommon and is about 1 in 3000 pregnancies. It can be due to adhesions or volvulus. It is usually characterized by short episodes of colicky pain, vomiting, and constipation. Clinical signs include abdominal tenderness and distention. Abdominal X-ray may be necessary if there is diagnostic difficulty. Treatment is by

fluid/electrolyte replacement and nasogastric suction, with surgical intervention rarely necessary. Think of this diagnosis in women with ongoing unexplained hyperemesis into the 2nd or 3rd trimester.

- Gastroenteritis: this common condition has many causes and can range from mild to severe. The usual symptoms are those of abdominal pain, vomiting, and diarrhoea. Dietary and travel history should be sought as well as and enquiry into symptoms in other family members. Examination reveals mild diffuse abdominal tenderness and borborygmi may be present. Bacterial and viral gastroenteritis is usually self-limiting. Dehydration can complicate the condition, and intravenous fluids and electrolyte supplementation may be necessary. If the condition does not resolve, consider other causes. Gastroenteritis may stimulate preterm labour. It is not known to cause any adverse perinatal outcomes.

- Peptic ulcer disease: this is rare in pregnancy, when the decreased gastric acid secretion is thought to reduce the incidence of this condition. Patients will often have a history of previous peptic ulceration or *H. pylori*, and typically present with epigastric or left upper quadrant burning pain that can radiate to the back. It is frequently relieved by food, antacids, or vomiting. Sudden onset of symptoms may indicate perforation, although this is rare in pregnancy, as is gastrointestinal bleeding. Epigastric tenderness is usually mild, but if perforation has occurred severe tenderness with signs of peritonitis may be present. H_2-receptor antagonists are usually sufficient to control symptoms, and testing and treatment for *H. pylori* should be performed after pregnancy.

- Inflammatory bowel disease (ulcerative colitis and Crohn's disease): this usually presents with abdominal pain and diarrhoea which can be accompanied by blood and mucus. Weight loss and anaemia are common. Exacerbations usually occur in the 1st and 2nd trimesters, and are more common in women who have active disease at the time of conception. Diagnosis can be confirmed by sigmoidoscopy and biopsy if necessary. Treatment with sulfasalazine and corticosteroids is safe in pregnancy, but the use of azathioprine should be avoided if possible. Surgical management may sometimes become necessary for bowel obstruction, perforation, intractable haemorrhage or toxic megacolon, and close liaison with the surgical team is essential.

- Diverticulitis: this is due to faecal material becoming trapped in the neck of diverticula allowing bacterial overgrowth. Although it is rare in pregnancy, up to a third of the population may have developed diverticula by the age of 45. Low left-sided pain is often accompanied by fever, nausea, and diarrhoea or constipation. Uncomplicated diverticulitis, will usually resolve with antibiotic treatment and food restriction. It can become complicated if perforation, abscesses or peritonitis develop, and this will require surgery.

Urinary tract
- Cystitis: this is common (1–2% of pregnancies) and causes suprapubic discomfort and tenderness. Dysuria is often absent, and asymptomatic bacteriuria is a risk factor. A mid-stream urine specimen culture will confirm the diagnosis. Treatment is with antibiotics. If untreated it may cause preterm labour or progress to pyelonephritis.
- Acute pyelonephritis: the patient feels unwell with fever, chills, nausea, vomiting, and dysuria. Uterine contractions may be present and if untreated the condition can lead to pre-term labour. Maternal and fetal tachycardia may accompany the fever, and examination reveals renal angle tenderness. A mid-stream specimen of urine should be collected for culture. Ward urinalysis should be taken and if it shows leucocytes, protein, and nitrites on dipstick examination, treatment is started with intravenous antibiotics, intravenous fluids, and analgesia. Recurrent episodes of pyelonephritis should be investigated with a renal ultrasound scan, and consideration given to prophylactic antibiotics.
- Urolithiasis: this occurs in about 1 in 500–2000 pregnancies. The symptoms of renal colic are severe intermittent flank pain which may radiate to the groin, and this is associated with nausea, vomiting, dysuria, and haematuria. Patients may give a history of recent or recurrent urinary tract infection, or of previous renal stones. The patient is often restless and unable to get comfortable, and palpation reveals tenderness of the renal angle, lower abdomen, or flank. Discussion of imaging with a radiologist is advisable: renal ultrasound should be the first line of investigation, and may show hydronephrosis or areas of calcification. If ultrasound is equivocal, a limited IVU may be necessary. The risk of radiation must be balanced against the risks of renal damage, preterm labour, or inappropriate treatment. Conservative management with intravenous fluids, antibiotics and analgesia will allow passage of the calculus in most cases. Surgical intervention may be required if conservative measures fail.

Other causes
- Sickle cell crises: these occur in about a third of women with sickle cell disease during pregnancy. Often no exacerbating factors other than pregnancy may be present. Most patients will have a diagnosis of sickle cell disease established before pregnancy. Abdominal pain can be a feature of sickling crises accompanied by worsening anaemia. Treatment of a crisis is by keeping patients well-hydrated, warm, and well oxygenated with adequate analgesia (a patient controlled morphine pump is often required). Early liaison with the haematology team is essential as blood transfusion and occasionally exchange transfusion are necessary. Delivery is for obstetric indications only, but if recurrent crises occur near term early elective delivery may be considered.
- Pleurisy: pulmonary embolism or pneumonia can result in pleurisy that can occasionally present as upper abdominal pain. These are considered in Chapter 2, pp. 38–40.

- Splenic infarction: this is a rare cause of abdominal pain and is usually associated with sickle cell disease. There is a large variation in symptomatology, with cases ranging from the clinically occult to severe left upper quadrant pain and maternal shock. In the latter, surgical management with partial or compete splenectomy is required.
- Malaria: this can present with abdominal pain. A travel history should be taken and a history of typical symptoms of headache, nausea, vomiting, chills, sweating, fever, fatigue, and muscular pains should be sought. A peripheral blood smear will demonstrate the presence of parasites. If the diagnosis is confirmed, seek specialist advice for management of the condition and choice of antimalarial therapy as the condition can rapidly deteriorate and lead to convulsions and even death.
- Acute intermittent porphyria: this is a rare genetic disorder more frequently manifest in women. Attacks can be precipitated by infections as well as drugs. The attack involves the innervation to the gut leading to abdominal pain which can radiate to the back. Urinary porphobilinogen is elevated. Treatment is supportive.
- Vascular complications: very rarely abdominal pain can be due to spontaneous rupture of intra-abdominal vessels such as the uterine or ovarian veins, or splenic or aortic aneurysms. Such cases will present with symptoms and signs of intra-abdominal bleeding and require laparotomy. Rectus sheath hematoma can occur due to rupture of the superior or inferior epigastric vessels or their branches. It usually causes sudden and severe abdominal pain. While usually self-limiting it can rarely expand leading to hypovolaemic shock, and requiring surgical intervention.

☠ Headache and feeling unwell

Headaches or generally feeling unwell are common complaints in pregnancy. Women with pre-existing migraine often improve in pregnancy, but migraine may first present in pregnancy. Before dismissing symptoms as being benign, more serious causes should be excluded by careful history and examination, including neurological assessment.

Associations

Symptoms of headache, feeling generally unwell, nausea and vomiting, confusion, impaired consciousness, and irrational behaviour frequently overlap. Such symptoms can be warning signs before a convulsion; indeed, many causes of convulsions can also cause such symptoms, and there is some overlap in the list of differential diagnosis with that of convulsions (see pp. 32–37).

Differential diagnosis

Diagnosis	Comments
Migraine	Difficult to distinguish from tension headache. Usually throbbing, unilateral, intensify over minutes, and may last for hours. History of prodromal symptoms ('aura'). Nausea and vomiting are common.
Cluster headaches	Unilateral. Nasal congestion and lacrimation are commonly associated. They occur in clusters, repeatedly every day, often for several weeks. The onset is sudden and typically start during sleep. Can be triggered by smoking, alcohol use, glare, and stress.
Tension headaches	These are due to muscular contractions of head and neck muscles. Dull, pressure-like headache which is usually worse at the scalp, temples, or back of the neck, are bilateral and described as 'a tight band on the head'. They are worsened or triggered by stress, fatigue, and noise, as well as by caffeine, alcohol, or tobacco use.
Pre-eclampsia	Patients seeking medical attention in severe pre-eclampsia are frequently triggered to seek help by headache or generally feeling unwell. The diagnosis is established by the findings of hypertension and proteinuria.

Differential diagnosis (Contd.)

Diagnosis	Comments
Infections: • Meningitis • Encephalitis • Cerebral abscess	History of non-specific prodromal illness is often present, with headaches typically evolving over hours or days. Pyrexia, neck stiffness and photophobia are often present, but petechial rash is only seen in meningococcal meningitis.
• Generalized sepsis	Frequently presents with headache and vague symptoms. Often accompanied by pyrexia. Efforts should be made to identify focus of infection before starting antibiotic treatment.
Cerebrovascular accidents: • Venous thrombosis • Infarction • Haemorrhage	Headache is severe and sudden in subarachnoid haemorrhage, and photophobia and altered conciousness is present in venous thrombosis. Focal neurological signs are often present. Imaging may not detect infarction in the first 24 hours. Venous sinus thrombosis is often due to underlying infection or pre-eclampsia.
Space occupying lesions: • Cerebral tumours	Progressive and severe headaches that are 'bursting' in nature and develop over days or weeks. May be associated with gradually worsening neurological impairment.
Metabolic/electrolyte imbalance: • Hypoglycaemia • Hyperglycaemia • Hyponatremia • Hypocalcemia	Causes of feeling unwell. Correction of the imbalance leads to improvement in symptoms. Can lead to convulsions if left untreated (see pp. 32–37).
Trauma	This will be evident from the history of head trauma.
Drugs or drug withdrawal: • Glyceryl trinitrate • Nifedipine	Used for tocolytic and antihypertensive treatment, both are commonly associated with headaches due to severe vasodilatation.
• Cocaine • Amphetamines • Alcohol	History of drug overdose, withdrawal or poison ingestion. A toxicology screen (urine/blood) should be performed if this is thought to be the underlying cause.

History

This should include onset (for example, gradual in tension headaches and migraine, rapid in vascular accidents); severity (typically very severe in subarachnoid haemorrhage); character (e.g. throbbing in migraine, band-like in tension headache); and site (e.g. unilateral in migraine, retro-orbital in cluster headaches). Precipitating factors should be sought and may include glare or light in migraines, cluster headaches, and meningitis. Associated symptoms may include neck stiffness in meningitis and vascular accidents; flashing lights or epigastric pain in pre-eclampsia; visual loss in glaucoma and temporal arteritis (both very rare causes of headaches in this age group); and neurological signs which may be of rapid onset in infectious and vascular complications, or of slow and progressive nature in space-occupying lesions.

Examination

- General: blood pressure will be elevated in pre-eclampsia and urine dipstick analysis demonstrate proteinuria. Pyrexia may indicate cerebral or generalized infection. Formal assessment of consciousness (using the Glasgow Coma Scale) should be performed, and signs of impaired consciousness should alert the clinician to possible intracranial pathology such as infection, vascular accidents, or space occupying lesions. Cerebral oedema may co-exist secondary to the above, but can also be a feature in pre-eclampsia.
- Neurological: detailed neurological examination should be performed and include fundoscopy which may reveal signs of raised intracranial pressure (papilloedema).

Investigations

These depend on the findings in the history and examination. A FBC may reveal leukocytosis in infection, and U&E will reveal electrolyte imbalance and both are useful in pre-eclampsia. In the presence of pyrexia blood cultures should be performed. Close liaison with neurology and radiology teams should be established to allow imaging of the brain using CT or MRI if there are any neurological signs. Lumbar puncture for the diagnosis of suspected meningitis/encephalitis should be performed after exclusion of increased intracranial pressure.

Treatment

Treatment will depend on the underlying cause. For tension and cluster headaches, as well as migraines, the mainstay therapy is simple analgesia such as paracetamol and codeine phosphate. Ergotamine should be avoided, and avoidance of triggers, such as smoking, alcohol use, specific foods should be advised. For cases with recurrent migraine resistant to treatment consideration should be given to prophylactic aspirin therapy.

☠ Convulsions in pregnancy

Convulsions in pregnancy are most commonly caused by epilepsy and eclampsia, and these are treated in more detail below. An unusual history, atypical symptoms and signs, or lack of response to treatment should alert one to the possibility of one of the rarer causes of convulsions in pregnancy, and these are listed in the differential diagnosis table, below.

Apart from convulsions, most of the conditions can present with non-specific symptoms, such as confusion, impaired consciousness or irrational behaviour, headache, nausea and vomiting. Accurate description of the convulsion will usually come from an observer. Careful examination, including a full neurological assessment is invaluable. Specialist input from the anaesthetic team, neurology, radiology and microbiology is essential.

Differential diagnosis of convulsions

Diagnosis	Comments
Eclampsia	Associated with hypertension and proteinuria
Epilepsy	Usually pre-existing history of epilepsy.
Infections: • Meningitis • Encephalitis • Cerebral malaria • Cerebral abscess	History of non-specific prodromal illness often present. Pyrexia, neck stiffness, and photophobia. Petechial rash in meningococcal meningitis only. Investigation: high inflammatory markers. In malaria positive blood film and anaemia. Lumbar puncture positive.
• Febrile convulsions	Identify focus of septicaemia. Intravenous antibiotics.
Cerebrovascular accidents: • Venous thrombosis • Infarction • Haemorrhage	Most cases post-natal. May have focal neurological signs prior to convulsion. Headache common (severe and sudden in subarachnoid haemorrhage), photophobia, and altered conciousness in venous thrombosis. Urgent CT or MRI, but infarction may appear normal in first 24 hours. Sinus thrombosis can also occur as a complication of infection or pre-eclampsia, and is treated with anticoagulation.
Space occupying lesions: • Cerebral tumours	Gradual, progressive neurological impairment. Imaging to identify lesion.

Differential diagnosis of convulsions (Contd.)

Diagnosis	Comments
Metabolic/electrolyte imbalance: • Hypoglycemia	Low glucose, responds to glucose treatment. Remember to seek cause for hypoglycaemia.
• Hyperglycaemia	High blood glucose, usually due to diabetic ketoacidosis. Responds to treatment.
• Hyponatremia	Low serum sodium. Look for causes of SIADH (Low serum osmolality High urine osmolality). Specialist treatment as possible myelolysis if rapid increase in sodium. Fluid restriction.
• Hypocalcemia	Causes include hypoparathyroidism and renal failure. Paraesthesia and tetany present. Serum calcium low, ECG abnormal (wide QT interval). Treat with calcium gluconate (cardiac monitoring).
Trauma	History of head trauma. Focal neurological findings. Imaging showing brain injury.
Drugs or drug withdrawal: • Cocaine • Amphetamines • Alcohol	History of drug overdose, withdrawal or poison ingestion. Toxicology screen (urine/blood) if suspicious of this.
Movement disorders or chorea	Usually evident from history.
Psychiatric disorders: • Psychogenic seizures • Pseudoseizures	Diagnosis of exclusion. Usually evident from history and clinical/negative laboratory findings.

General management of seizures

The general management of seizures is given here. Subsequent management will depend on the underlying cause, as given in the differential diagnosis above. As the majority of convulsions in pregnancy are caused by epilepsy and eclampsia, these are described in more detail below. Remember that unusual history, symptoms or signs as well as failure of treatment may be due to a rarer cause of convulsions.

1. **Call for assistance**—senior obstetrician and anaesthetist.
2. **Protect the patient**—avoid maternal trauma by placing the patient in a safe environment.
3. **ABC**—assess **A**irway, **B**reathing and **C**irculation. Measurement of blood pressure and testing for proteinuria should exclude eclampsia.
4. **Respiratory support**—give oxygen.
5. **Intravenous access**
6. **Bloods**—draw blood for FBC, U&E, liver function, glucose, clotting, G&S.
7. **Glucose**—give 50 ml of glucose (50%) if hypoglycaemia suspected.
8. **Assess fetal heart rate**

9. **Abolish seizures**—drugs used depend on the cause (see below). In summary:
   Epilepsy
   - Lorazepam 0.1 mg/kg IV (2 mg/min)
   - Repeat at 10 min
       or
     - Diazepam 10 mg IV bolus
     - Repeat at 10 min 2 mg
   - 10–20 mg **rectally** if no IV access
   Eclampsia
   - Loading dose magnesium sulphate 4 g/40 ml IV (over 10 min)
   - Maintenance dose magnesium sulphate 1 g/10 ml/hour
   - If recurrent seizures, further boluses of magnesium sulphate 2 g IV
   - If magnesium contraindicated, give diazepam 10 mg IV bolus
10. **Control blood pressure**
11. **Consider delivery**—depending on the underlying cause, seizure activity, gestational age, and fetal well-being.
12. **Establish a cause**—if this is the first seizure, investigations are required after the acute event and should include specialist neurological assessment, FBC, U&E, LFTs, glucose and calcium, imaging (MRI or CT scan), and in some cases EEG or lumbar puncture.
13. **Debrief prior to discharge**—ensure that prior to discharge the patient understands their diagnosis, seizure safety, driving regulations, and that adequate follow-up is made.

Epilepsy

Background

Although epileptic convulsions during pregnancy carry a high risk to both mother and fetus, many women will discontinue their anticonvulsant treatment due to fears over fetal abnormalities. This, in addition to increased metabolism and excretion of anticonvulsants and changes in intravascular volume and binding proteins, means that seizure frequency increases in up to a third of cases. Suitable antenatal care should include careful management of anticonvulsant therapy in order to minimize the risk of seizures, using the lowest effective dose of anticonvulsants possible. Apart from tailoring and modifying anticonvulsant medication, pregnancy care should include high-dose folic acid periconceptually, detailed ultrasound, and (in women taking enzyme-inducing antiepileptic drugs) oral vitamin K from around 36 weeks of gestation. Labour and delivery is best in a consultant-led maternity unit and seizure prophylaxis should be considered for high-risk cases. There is no contraindication to normal vaginal delivery. Caesarean section may be performed for obstetric reasons.

Most patients will have a pre-existing history of epilepsy but in some instances this may be their first seizure. In these cases a full work-up, including specialist neurological assessment, FBC, U&E, liver function tests, glucose and calcium, imaging (MRI or CT scan), and EEG is required after the acute event.

Risks of seizures
- Maternal
  - Trauma
  - Aspiration
  - Abruption
  - Status epilepticus.
- Fetal
  - Hypoxia
  - Abruption.

Management

1–8 The first 8 steps are given under the general management of seizures. Eclampsia as a cause should be excluded by checking BP and urine for proteinuria. Then steps 9 onwards are undertaken.

9. **Abolish seizures**
   - Lorazepam 0.1 mg/kg IV (2 mg/min)
                    or
   - Diazepam 10 mg IV bolus, followed by 2 mg boluses if required
                    or
   - Diazepam 10–20 mg can be given rectally if no intravenous access
   - If seizures continue
   - Phenytoin 15 mg/kg IV (maximum rate 50 mg/min) with ECG monitoring

10. **If seizures continue** (refractory status epilepticus)
    - Inform HDU/ITU (anticipate need for ventilation)
    - Prepare for delivery (see step 11)
    - Seek specialist advice
    - Consider third-line drugs (some are unlicenced)
      - Phenobarbitone 10 mg/kg IV (maximum rate 100 mg/min)
      - Propofol 1–2 mg/kg loading, then 3–10 mg/kg/hour
      - Midazolam 0.2 mg/kg loading, then 0.06–1.1 mg/kg/hour
      - Thiopentone
    - Consider other causes
      - Eclampsia
      - Meningitis/encephalitis
      - Trauma
      - Drugs

11. **When to deliver** depends on seizure activity, gestational age and fetal wellbeing.
    - If seizures are controlled, continue with appropriate pregnancy or labour care.
    - Intractable/recurrent generalized seizures during labour or in the late 3rd trimester may require Caesarean section under general anaesthetic.

12. Ensure **vitamin K** is given to the neonate.

Eclampsia

Background

Pre-eclampsia/eclampsia are multi-system disorders that can progress rapidly with high risks to mother and fetus. Women with eclampsia may have been known to have pre-eclampsia in their current pregnancy, and there is little diagnostic difficulty. Frequently, it is the symptoms of fulminant pre-eclampsia or eclampsia that trigger admission. Convulsions due to eclampsia with apparently mild or delayed onset of hypertension and proteinuria are widely reported. Predisposing factors include chronic hypertension, renal disease or diabetes; multiple pregnancy; thrombophilia; or abnormal uterine artery Doppler in mid-gestation. Over a third of eclamptic fits occur postnatally.

The aims of management are:
- To arrest and prevent convulsions
- To control blood pressure
- To effect planned, timely and safe delivery.

Risks of seizures
- Maternal:
  - Trauma
  - Aspiration
  - Haemolysis, elevated liver enzymes, low platelets (HELLP syndrome)
  - Pulmonary oedema
  - Cerebrovascular accidents
  - Abruption
  - Anaesthetic and surgical complications of delivery.
- Fetal:
  - Iatrogenic premature delivery
  - Hypoxia
  - Abruption.

Management
1–8 The first 8 steps are given under the general management of seizures. Eclampsia as a cause should be excluded by checking BP and urine for proteinuria. Then steps 9 onwards are undertaken.

9. Start HDU chart with 5 minutely BP and pulse until seizures arrested and BP controlled

10. Abolish seizures
- Loading dose magnesium sulphate 4 g/40 ml IV (over 10 min)
- Maintenance dose magnesium sulphate 1 g/10 ml/hour
- If recurrent seizures, further boluses of magnesium sulphate 2 g IV
- or increase maintenance to 1.5–2 g/hour
- If magnesium is contraindicated give diazepam 10 mg IV bolus

11. Pre-load circulation with colloid—250 ml gelofusine IV/20 min.

12. Antihypertensive treatment
- Labetalol 200 mg/100 ml IV at 20 mg/hour
- Double every 30 min until target BP reached

  or
- Hydralazine 5 mg IV (1 mg/min)
- Repeat after 15 min if SBP>160; DBP >110 or MAP >125
- If after 3 boluses SBP>160; DBP >110 or MAP >125 start hydralazine infusion: hydralazine 40 mg/40 ml IV

Titrate to maternal BP:

Start	2.4 ml/h (40 µg/min)
30 min	4.8 ml/h (80 µg/min)
60 min	7.2 ml/h (120 µg/min)
90 min	9.6 ml/h (160 µg/min)

Reduce by 1.2 ml/h if appropriate

If the pulse rate >140/min or there is a contraindication to hydralazine, give labetalol:

or

- Oral treatment with nifedipine MR/retard 10 mg, swallowed whole, may be possible in certain cases
- This can be repeated at 2 hours if needed.

13. **When to deliver:** delivery should be timed and well-planned, after control of seizures and blood pressure has been achieved. Uncontrolled hypertension or ongoing seizures make delivery inappropriate. Always ensure that:
    - The maternal condition is stable
    - Senior personnel are present

    In the presence of eclampsia, delivery is usually by Caesarean section, preferably with epidural or spinal anaesthetic. If thrombocytopaenia or coagulation disorder is present, general anaesthesia may be necessary. After 34 weeks of gestation, and if the condition is well controlled, induction of labour may be considered if the cervix is favourable.

14. **Third stage:** oxytocin bolus. Avoid ergometrine or syntometrine as this can cause hypertension. If possible avoid an oxytocin infusion as this can cause pulmonary oedema.

15. **After delivery**
    - HDU care, consider central venous pressure line early
    - Careful monitoring of pulse/BP/SpO$_2$
    - Continue seizure prophylaxis for 24 hours after last seizure or delivery
    - Antihypertensive as required
    - Fluid balance: fluid restriction to 85 ml/h with hourly urine output measurement.

:☠: Chest pain in pregnancy

Definition
A pain arising from inside the chest wall.

Nature
Constricting suggests angina, oesophageal reflux, or anxiety. A sharp pain suggests origin from the pleura or pericardium. A prolonged (>30 min), dull, central crushing pain suggests MI.

Radiation
To shoulder, either or both arms, or neck/jaw suggests cardiac ischaemia. Epigastric pain may be cardiac.

Precipitants
Pain associated with cold, exercise, palpitations, or emotions suggest cardiac pain or anxiety. If brought on by food, alcohol, or position consider reflux. Prolonged bed rest, DVT, thrombophilia, venous stasis, recent air flight, age, parity, drugs, sickle cell disease, and recent surgery suggest PE. Smoking, upper respiratory tract infection, immunosuppression, pre-existing lung disease, recent contact with birds, and drugs (e.g. steroids) may predispose to pneumonia.

Associations
Dyspnoea is a common association. Myocardial infarction may also cause nausea, vomiting, and sweating.

Causes
- Cardiac
  - Angina[1]
  - Myocardial infarction.[2]
- Non-cardiac
  - Reflux oesophagitis[3]
  - Anxiety
  - PE[1]
  - Pneumonia.[4]

Diagnostic steps
- Full history should include: nature, radiation, precipitating factors and associations. Abdominal pain may suggest pelvic vein thrombosis or diaphragmatic irritation. Breathlessness is more common in PE and pneumonia. Syncope can occur in large PE. Cough is a common symptom in PE and pneumonia. Purulent sputum and fever with rigors are suggestive of pneumonia. Vomiting and bradycardia may result from vagal effect in MI. Past medical, family, and drug history is useful.
- Physical examination: vital signs (blood pressure [hypotension in PE and MI], pulse rate and nature, pyrexia [can occur in MI, pneumonia and PE], cyanosis [PE]), Third heart sound, parasternal heave and elevated JVP suggestive of right-sided cardiac failure is more common in PE, pericardial rub, and secondary effects in MI. Check respiratory systems for signs and legs for evidence of DVT.
- Relief with oxygen, GTN—?cardiac origin.

Investigations

- ECG—look for evidence of MI. $S_1Q_3T_3$ may be normal in pregnancy
- Chest X-ray
- C-reactive protein
- Troponin I
- Glutamic acid transaminases
- Creatinine phosphokinase (MB isoenzyme)
- Blood cultures
- Arterial blood gases
- Echocardiography
- Ventilation perfusion scan
- Dopplers/venogram for pelvis/lower limbs.
- Impedance plethysmography & thermography
- Spiral computed tomography (CT)
- MRI.

Management

- Multi-disciplinary management with the obstetrician anaesthetist and relevant medical sub-specialist e.g. cardiologist, respiratory physician.
- Symptomatic relief with oxygen, propped up position.
- Pain relief with opiates.
- Fetal monitoring.
- Obstetric plan of management including the possible need for delivery.
- Treat specific illness:
  - intravenous heparin, thrombolytic agents and surgical thrombo-lectomy in PE. IVC filter may be inserted in recurrent emboli[5]. Thrombolytic agents although unlicensed may be used if necessary in PE.
  - managed in a CCU setting with nitroglycerine, aspirin, thrombolytic agents and other necessary drugs.
  - paracetamol and tepid sponging to reduce the complications of pyrexia. Antibiotic usage to be managed with microbiologist.
  - H_2 receptor antagonists and/or antacids and dietary advice may relieve reflux oesophagitis.

Differentiating signs and symptoms

Symptom/sign	MI	PE	Pneumonia
Sputum	Dry	Dry	Productive
Abd pain	–	+	±
Lungs	Crepts	–	Ronchi
Heart sounds	Quiet 1st 3rd HS	3rd HS	N
BP	↓ or N	↓ or N	N
Pulse	Thready, low vol	N	N
Pulse rate		↑ or N	↑ or N

N = No change

Differences in common investigations

Investigation	MI	PE	Pneumonia
CXR	N	Usually N/ Wedge-shaped infarction, pleural effusion, atelectasis, areas of translucency in underperfused lung	Patchy/ consolidation
ECG	Varied	N/ right axis deviation, right bundle branch block, peaked waves in lead II, S1 Q3 T3 pattern	N
Echo	Reduced function	Right-sided strain	N

N = No change

References

1. Graves CR (2002). Acute pulmonary complications during pregnancy. *Clin Obstet Gynecol*, **45**(2), 369–76.
2. Nelson-Piercy C (2002). Respiratory disease. In Handbook of obstetric medicine, 2nd edition (ed C. Nelson-Piercy). London: Martin Dunitz, pp. 59–81.
3. Shehata HA, Nelson-Piercy C (2001). Medical diseases complicating pregnancy. *Anaes Intern Care Med*, **2**(6), 225–33.
4. Roth A, Elkayam U (1996). Acute myocardial infarction associated with pregnancy. *Ann Intern Med*, 1:**25**(9), 751–62.
5. Royal College of Obstetricians and Gynaecologists (2001). *Thromboembolic Disease in Pregnancy and the Puerperium: Acute Management*. Guideline No. 28. London.

☠ Breathlessness/difficulty in breathing/chest discomfort

Definition (dyspnoea)

It is the subjective sensation of shortness of breath, often exacerbated by exertion. Fifty per cent of pregnant women are aware of breathlessness before 20 weeks gestation. It reaches the maximum incidence at 28–31 weeks gestation.

Precipitants

Prolonged bed rest, DVT, thrombophilia, venous stasis, recent air flight, age, parity, drugs and recent surgery may suggest PE. Smoking, URTI and immunosuppression may predispose to pneumonia. Allergens, cold air, emotions, infection, drugs, exercise, and stress are related to asthma.

Associations

Exertional dyspnoea, orthopnoea, paroxysmal nocturnal dyspnoea, and peripheral oedema are associated with cardiac failure. There is usually an underlying cause leading to cardiac failure. Acid reflux, polyarteritis nodosa, Churg–Strauss syndrome, and other atopic diseases have known associations with asthma.

Causes of breathlessness

Acute	Sub acute	Chronic
• Hyperventilation/anxiety	• Asthma	• Physiological
• Acute asthma	• Lung parenchymal	• Anaemia
• PE	disease	• Chronic lung
• Acute pulmonary	e.g. pneumonia,	disease
oedema	alveolitis,	• Cardiac causes
• Foreign body	effusions	• Mitral stenosis
• Pneumothorax		• Puerperal
		cardiomyopathy

Diagnostic steps

- Full history: abdominal pain may suggest pelvic vein thrombosis or diaphragmatic irritation. Syncope can occur in large PE. Cough is a common symptom in PE and pneumonia but mainly nocturnal in cardiac failure and asthma. Purulent sputum, rigors are suggestive of pneumonia. Tachypnoea, audible wheeze, and hyper inflated chest are noted in asthma. Consider acquired cardiac lesions such as mitral stenosis in immigrant women from Africa, Middle East, and Asia. Past medical, family, and drug history are important.
- Physical examination—vital signs (blood pressure [hypotension in PE, hypotension and narrow pulse pressure in cardiac failure], pulse rate [pulsus alterans and tachycardia in cardiac failure] and nature, pyrexia [can occur in pneumonia and PE] cyanosis [PE, cardiac failure]), cardiac

sounds (3rd heart sound, parasternal heave and ↑ JVP suggestive of right-sided cardiac failure is more common in PE; ↑ JVP, hepatomegaly, cardiomegaly, gallop rhythm, murmurs in cardiac failure); respiratory systems (pleural effusion, bilateral basal crepts, wheeze and tachypnoea in cardiac failure; polyphonic wheeze, diminished air entry or silent chest in asthma); and legs for evidence of DVT.

Investigations

- Peak flow meter
- Pulse oximetry
- ECG—$S_1Q_3T_3$ may be normal in pregnancy.
- Chest X-ray
- Troponin I
- B-type natriuretic peptide
- Blood and sputum cultures
- Arterial blood gases
- Echocardiography
- C-reactive protein—non-specific, suggestive of inflammatory process
- Spirometry
- Ventilation perfusion scan
- Dopplers/venogram for pelvis/ lower limbs.
- Impedance plethysmography & thermography
- Spiral CT
- MRI

Management

- Multi-disciplinary management with the obstetrician, anaesthetist and relevant medical sub-specialist e.g. cardiologist, respiratory physician.
- Symptomatic relief with oxygen, propped up position.
- Pain relief with opiates.
- Fetal monitoring.
- Obstetric plan of management including the need for delivery.
- Treat specific illness:
  - *PE:* intravenous heparin, thrombolytic agents, and surgical thrombo- lectomy in PE. IVC filter may be inserted in recurrent emboli.
  - *Pneumonia:* paracetamol and tepid sponging to reduce the complications of pyrexia. Antibiotic usage to be managed with microbiologist.
  - *Cardiac:* treat exacerbating factors e.g. anaemia, thyroid disease, infection. Avoid exacerbating factors e.g. NSAIDS (fluid retention), verapamil (negative inotrope). Stop smoking. Reduce salt intake. Maintain optimal weight and nutrition.
    Cardiac—use appropriate drugs e.g. diuretics, spironolactone, ACE-inhibitor, β-blockers, digoxin, vasodilators. Heart transplant is final option.
  - *Asthma:* in severe acute attacks, salbutamol in nebulizer, oral steroids, and intravenous aminophylline. Managed in ITU if intubation is expected. Possible use of $MgSO_4$. Revert to $β_2$-agonist and steroid inhalers when stable.
  - Physiological cause is a diagnosis of exclusion.

Differentiating signs and symptoms

Symptom/sign	Cardiac failure	Asthma	PE	Pneumonia
Sputum	Nocturnal	Nocturnal	Dry	Productive
Abd pain	–	–	+	±
Lungs	Bibasilar crepts	Exp ronchi ↓ air entry/ Silent	–	Ronchi
Heart sounds	Gallop rhythm	N	3rd HS	N
BP	Low	N	↓/N	N
Pulse—character	↓ volume, pulsus alterans	Pulsus paradoxus	N	N
Pulse rate	↑	↑/N	↑/N	↑/N

N = No change

Differences in common investigations

Investigation	Cardiac failure	Asthma	PE	Pneumonia
CXR	Hilar shadowing, Kerley B lines, cardiomegaly, pleural effusion	Hyperinflated lungs	N/Wedge-shaped infarction, pleural effusion, atelectasis, areas of translucency in underperfused lung	Patchy/consolidation
ECG	Left ventricular strain/enlargement	N	N/ right axis deviation, right bundle branch block, peaked waves in lead II	N
Echo	Cardiomegaly, ↓ function, ± valve abnormally	N	Right-sided strain	N

N = No change

Recommended reading

1. Nelson-Piercy C (2002). Handbook of obstetric medicine, 2nd edition. London: Martin Dunitz, 284–285.
2. Graves CR (2002). Acute pulmonary complications during pregnancy. *Clin Obstet Gynecol* **45**(2) 369–76.
3. Bhide A, Shehata H-A (2004). Respiratory disease in pregnancy. *Current Obstetrics and Gynaecology,* **14**(3), 175–182.
4. Greer IA, ed. (1997). Thromboembolic Disease in Obstetrics and Gynaecology. *Baillières Clin Obstet Gynaeco,* **11**, 431–45.
5. Report on Confidential Enquiry into Maternal Deaths in the United Kingdom 1994–96. London: HMSO, 1998.
6. Royal College of Obstetricians and Gynaecologists. Report of the RCOG Working Party on Prophylaxis against Thromboembolism in Gynaecology and Obstetrics. London: Chameleon Press, 1995.
7. Royal College of Obstetricians and Gynaecologists. Thromboembolic Disease in Pregnancy and the Puerperium: Acute Management. Guideline No. 28. London. April 2001.

⑦ Jaundice

Jaundice is the clinical manifestation of raised bilirubin levels in blood. Jaundice is detectable clinically at bilirubin concentrations of 30 μmol/L. The haem component of spent red blood cells is normally broken down to bilirubin (predominantly in the spleen and bone marrow) and transported to the liver bound to albumin. In the liver the bilirubin is conjugated making it water-soluble and then it is excreted in bile. The level of conjugated bilirubin in blood is normally very low. Bacterial action in the bowel converts conjugated bilirubin to urobilinogen, some of which is oxidized to stercobilin, which in turn gives the brown colour to normal faeces. Some urobilinogen is reabsorbed, passing to the liver in the portal blood and re-excreted in the bile thus completing the so-called enterohepatic recirculation. A small proportion of the urobilinogen is excreted in the urine, having escaped into the systemic circulation.

Hyperbilirubinaemia is thus a consequence of either excessive production of bilirubin (usually extrahepatic causes such as haemolysis) or inadequate hepatic capacity to eliminate normal amounts of bilirubin through liver injury, congenital deficiency of enzymes, or an obstruction in the elimination pathway from the liver (obstructive jaundice).

Main causes of jaundice in pregnancy

- Unique to pregnancy
  - intrahepatic cholestasis of pregnancy
  - acute fatty liver of pregnancy
  - hyperemesis gravidarum
  - HELLP syndrome
- Coincidental to pregnancy
  - Viral hepatitis
  - Gallstone disease (cholelithiasis)
  - Congenital disorders of bilirubin metabolism
  - Autoimmune hepatitis
  - Cirrhosis
  - Neoplasia.

Intrahepatic cholestasis of pregnancy

Also referred to simply as 'cholestasis of Pregnancy'. Commonly presents with itching in the 3rd trimester of pregnancy.

Clinical features

- Severe itching/pruritus affecting trunk and limbs but no visible rash even if there are excoriations.
- There may be associated malaise and insomnia.
- On direct questioning there may be dark urine, anorexia, and malabsorption of fat leading to steatorrhoea.
- Raised bile acids and often abnormal liver function tests.
- A positive family history in up to half the patients suggesting an autosomal dominant inheritance pattern.
- An episode where a similar syndrome was precipitated by the administration of exogenous oestrogens such as the combined oral contraceptive pill (COCP).

Laboratory findings

- Raised bile acids (may be the only biochemical abnormality)
- Moderate elevation in ALT
- Raised alkaline phosphatase (above normal pregnancy values)
- Raised bilirubin
- Raised γGT.

Maternal risks

Vitamin K deficiency and increased risk of PPH.

Fetal risks

Significant risk of intrauterine fetal death, spontaneous preterm delivery, intrapartum fetal distress, meconium stained liquor. The risk of stillbirth increases towards term and is greatest after 37 weeks but does not correlate to maternal symptoms.

Management

- Counselling regarding fetal risks, for close fetal surveillance until delivery at 37–38 weeks.
- Fetal surveillance by a combination of fetal activity monitoring by the mother as well as regular ultrasound scans to monitor fetal growth and amniotic fluid index and cardiotocography.
- Maternal monitoring by regular LFTs, bile acids and coagulation screening.
- Maternal vitamin K supplementation with an oral dose 10 mg daily to reduce the risks of maternal and fetal bleeding.
- Pruritus can be symptomatically treated with antihistamines such as terfenadine, chlorpheniramine, or promethazine. Ursodeoxycholic acid (UDCA) provides impressive relief of pruritus and improvement in both bile acid levels and LFTs. The dosage is 8–12 mg/kg per day in 2 divided doses.

Postnatal management

Monitoring of biochemical resolution is essential but if diagnosis is suspect or condition appears to be progressive further invasive investigation in the form of a liver biopsy may be indicated.

The recurrence in future pregnancies is 50%. Women should be counselled to avoid the combined oral contraceptive but HRT appears to be safe.

Acute fatty liver of pregnancy (AFLP)

This is a rare complication occurring in pregnancy, with an approximate incidence of 1 in 10 000. There appears to be an association with maternal obesity, male fetus (three times more common) and multiple pregnancy. There is considerable overlap with HELLP syndrome and AFLP may be a variant of pre-eclampsia.

Clinical features

- Gradual onset malaise, nausea and anorexia after 30 weeks gestation and often approaching term.
- Severe vomiting and abdominal pain.
- Jaundice within 2 weeks of onset of symptoms.

- Ascites with developing signs and symptoms of liver failure with hepatic encephalopathy, DIC, and renal failure.
- Hypertension and proteinuria in 50% of cases.
- Extreme polydipsia or pseudodiabetes insipidus.

Laboratory findings
- Abnormal LFTs with significant elevation in transaminases and alkaline phosphatase.
- Profound hypoglycaemia.
- Marked hyperuricemia, out of proportion to other features of pre-eclampsia.
- Blood film is often leukemoid or may show leukoerythroblastic change.
- Gold standard for diagnosis is liver biopsy with special fat stains (histology: microvesicular steatosis) but not practical or necessary in pregnancy.
- Liver imaging by US, CT, or MRI may show evidence of fat infiltration but may also appear normal.

Maternal risks
Fulminant hepatic failure, hepatic encephalopathy, coagulopathy, death.

Fetal/neonatal risks
Intrauterine fetal death with a perinatal mortality rate of 15–65%. Neonatal risks include transient derangement in LFTs and hypoglycaemia.

Management
- Maternal resuscitation and stabilization.
- Continuous fetal monitoring.
- Urgent delivery.
- Admit to intensive care or high dependency area and multidisciplinary input from obstetrician, physician, and anaesthetist.
- Vaginal delivery probably better if feasible in view of potential to develop coagulation problems.
- GA may be safer than regional technique for Caesarean section. Must have low threshold for drains.
- Parenteral glucose to maintain euglycemia.
- Neomycin and lactulose to decolonize the bowel, reducing ammonia production.
- Multivitamin supplementation.
- In fulminant hepatic failure, transfer to regional liver unit and possible liver transplantation.

Postnatal
Gradual return to normal liver function. If abnormal LFTs persist beyond 6 weeks consider alternative pathologies. Recurrence risk is in the region of 20% in subsequent pregnancy. Close surveillance of LFTs with use of OCP is recommended.

Hyperemesis gravidarum
Onset in the 1st trimester of severe or protracted vomiting causing fluid and electrolyte imbalance, weight loss of approximately 3 kg and necessitating hospital admission. Occurs in 0.5–1% of pregnancies.

Investigations

Hyperemesis is a diagnosis of exclusion and investigations serve to identify any underlying causes and guide treatment.

- FBC may reveal raised haematocrit and abnormally raised white cell count.
- U&E. Hyperemesis is associated with hyponatraemia, hypokalaemia, and a hypochloraemic metabolic alkalosis. Serum urea is low due to low protein intake, but an elevated urea to creatinine ratio may be a further indication of dehydration.
- LFTs serve as a marker of severity of the hyperemesis. Deranged LFTs in the most severe cases (30–50%).
- Thyroid function tests may reveal a picture of biochemical thyrotoxicosis with a clinically euthyroid patient.
- Urinalysis may reveal ketonuria and an MSU needs to be sent to rule out UTI as cause for vomiting.
- Pelvic ultrasound scan, to confirm a viable singleton intrauterine pregnancy as both multiple pregnancy and molar pregnancy are associated with hyperemesis.

Maternal risks

- Deficiency of cyanocobalamin (B12) and pyridoxine (B6) causing anaemia and peripheral neuropathy.
- Wernicke's encephalopathy (WE) which can lead to maternal death. WE is due to thiamine deficiency (Vit B1). Symptoms of WE include diplopia, abnormal ocular movements, ataxia, and confusion. Typical ocular signs are nystagmus, gaze palsy and 6th cranial nerve palsy. There is a higher incidence of abnormal LFTs in patients with hyperemesis gravidarum complicated by WE compared to patients with hyperemesis alone. Confirmation of the diagnosis is by detecting reduced red cell transketolase activity or elevated thiamine pyrophosphate activity. There are characteristic lesions around the aqueduct and fourth ventricle on MRI scanning.
- Persistent prolonged vomiting may lead to haematemesis due to oesophageal Mallory–Weiss tear.
- Development of a catabolic state with weight loss, muscle wasting, and weakness.
- Rarely, total parenteral nutrition may be required via central venous pressure line.
- Hyponatraemia with plasma Na <120 mmol/L may lead to lethargy, seizures, and respiratory arrest along with risks of central pontine myelinolysis from rapid reversal of severe hyponatraemia.

Fetal risks

- No increase in congenital abnormalities.
- In severe hyperemesis in mother with significant weight loss (>5%), infants likely to have lower birth weights and birth weight percentiles.
- If maternal WE supervenes, significant risk (up to 40%) of fetal death.

Management
- Early aggressive rehydration. Avoid dextrose containing fluids as it may precipitate WE or worsen hyponatraemia. Titrate IV fluids against daily measurement of electrolytes.
- Regular urinalysis to monitor ketonuria, as symptoms of hyperemesis are worsened by ketosis. Breaking the cycle of nausea/vomiting, starvation, and ketosis is needed to prevent further exacerbation of nausea and vomiting.
- Antiemetics such as metoclopramide, prochloperazine, promethazine. In intractable cases ordansetron has also been used. In its severest and prolonged forms, hyperemesis gravidarum can be treated by a regime of intravenous hydrocortisone. If response is obtained follow on with oral prednisolone. Involvement of a dietician is helpful in these rare but challenging cases.
- Where LFTs are abnormal or the course has been protracted, supplementation with vitamins such as thiamine is recommended (25–50 mg tds orally, or 100 mg IV infusion in 100 ml saline).
- Anti-gastroesophageal reflux measures may also help in the form of elevation of the head of the bed, small frequent and bland meals, aliginates and H_2 receptor antagonists such as ranitidine.
- Psychological support and reassurance is essential.
- Total parenteral nutrition may be required very rarely.
- In intractable cases termination of pregnancy needs to be considered.

Viral hepatitis

Commonest cause of hepatic dysfunction in pregnancy is viral hepatitis.

Hepatitis A
- Faecal–oral transmission, inversely related to levels of sanitation.
- Short incubation of 14–50 days.
- Clinical features: abrupt but non-specific clinical features of flu-like illness, nausea, anorexia, vomiting, diarrhoea, fatigue. Cholestatic jaundice with pale stools, dark urine and pruritus follows prodromal illness. Usually a self-limiting illness.
- Management and prognosis similar to non-pregnant women.
- Post-exposure immunoprophylaxis may not prevent viral shedding. Potentially infected individuals should be isolated.
- Asymptomatic women in the 3rd trimester in contact with an index case should be given immunoglobulin (increased risks of preterm labour), as should women about to travel to high prevalence areas.

Hepatitis B
- DNA virus with incubation period 2–6 months but detectable in circulation from 1 month post infection,
- Main routes of transmission are blood and blood products, IV drug abuse, sexual activity. Vertical transmission is the predominant route in developing world.
- Clinical features: in acute HBV infection, approximately two-thirds are asymptomatic, subclinical, or associated with minimal, influenza-like symptoms. There may be upper gastrointestinal symptoms such as nausea, vomiting, anorexia, right hypochondrial discomfort but no

evidence of jaundice in almost half the cases. May however be followed by a protracted period of malaise and anorexia.

- Prognosis: complete resolution in 90% of cases within 6 months. Remaining 10% become chronic carriers where HbsAg persists for over 6 months with symptoms (chronic active hepatitis—CAH) or without symptoms but deranged LFTs (chronic persistent hepatitis—CPH). Rarely infection may progress to fulminant infection, hepatic failure, and death.
- Diagnosis: through detection of viral specific antigens and antibodies. HbsAg is an antigen from the viral capsule and indicates infectivity. Anti Hbs antibody is an antibody to the surface antigen and a marker of immunological response and cure. HbeAg is the antigen from the core of the virus and indicates high infectivity and high risk of vertical transmission (90% risk). Presence of Hbe antibody, which is the antibody to core antigen, indicates partial immunological response and low risk of transmission (10%).
- Management: symptomatic and supportive to control nausea and vomiting. Monitor hydration, uterine activity, and LFTs. Counselling, testing, and vaccination of family members and sexual contacts. No congenital syndrome or risk of teratogenesis.
- Obstetric significance: vertical transmission carries a 90% risk of chronic active or chronic persistent hepatitis hence justifying universal antenatal screening. Majority of infants are infected at time of birth from blood and body fluids with a small proportion through transplacental bleeds in utero. Antenatal detection of HbsAg should therefore be followed with a preventative program of active and passive immunization at birth. This involves the newborn receiving hepatitis B immune globulin (Hblg) IM within 12 hours of birth along with the first of 3 doses of recombinant vaccine in the other thigh. The 2nd and 3rd doses should be administered at 1 and 6 months and immunity confirmed at one year.

Hepatitis C

- Commonest cause of post transfusion hepatitis, with 50–90% of IV drug abusers (IVDA) in UK being HCV infected.
- Significant risk (60–80%) of chronic infection, with detection of HCV antibody being a marker of persistent infection. Cirrhosis and primary hepatocellular cancer are associated with chronic HCV infection.
- Routes of transmission are blood and blood products, sexual activity and IV drug use. Vertical transmission is affected by viral load and co-infection with HIV. Higher risk of vertical transmission if mother positive for HCV RNA as well as anti-HCV antibody but in chronic HCV infection, level of transaminases does not affect rates of transmission. Transmission through breast milk is uncommon.
- No vaccines to prevent HCV infection and HCV immune globulin is not recommended to infants of HCV positive mothers.
- Treatment with alpha interferon may lead to biochemical, histological, and virological improvement in 25% of patients after 6–12 months therapy but interferons are contraindicated in pregnancy.

Hepatitis E
- Predominantly waterborne, non-A, non-B form of enteric hepatitis.
- Epidemics associated with contaminated water in India, Southeast Asia (Nepal, Burma), North Africa (Ethiopia), and Middle East.
- Antibody immunoassays available in reference centers and can distinguish acute infection (IgM) from previous exposure (IgG).
- Not reported in UK except in travellers returning from high prevalence areas.
- Clinical features are similar to Hepatitis A and are self-limiting so supportive care.
- The obstetric significance is that the virus appears to have a predilection for pregnant women—reason unknown.
- Infection in pregnancy especially if acquired in the 3rd trimester is associated with increased maternal mortality.
- No immunoprophylaxis available.

Hepatitis—other viral causes

Epstein–Barr (EBV)
- Common transmission routes include sexual contact and via body fluids such as saliva.
- Blood borne transmission uncommon.
- Commonest form is in young adults and children—infectious mononucleosis (glandular fever).
- No special predilection for pregnancy.
- Less than 5% of cases develop hepatitis.

Cytomegalovirus (CMV)
- May account for up to 10% of mental retardation in children up to 6 years of age.
- Risk of primary infection in pregnancy is 1–2%.
- Amongst women of childbearing age 50–80% are seropositive for CMV.
- Routes of transmission are sexual contact, through transfused blood and perinatally either transplacentally or from exposure to the virus from the cervix or birth canal.
- After primary infection, the virus persists and latent virus reactivation may occur in 3–5% of women during pregnancy.
- Majority of infections are asymptomatic or associated with malaise, fever, atypical lymphocytosis and lymphopenia with hepatitis being a rare complication.
- Diagnosis of primary infection is by detecting a significant rise in IgM levels (persists for 4–8 months) with a recurrent infection heralded by a rise in IgG levels.
- Primary maternal infection carries up to 40% risk of fetal infection.
- CMV is found in 1% of newborns of whom 5–10% are clinically affected at birth and a further 5–10% develop long-term sequelea. Thus 85% of babies born to women with CMV in pregnancy, including 75% of infected infants have no CMV related problems at birth or thereafter.
- Confirmation of CMV infection in pregnancy has to be accompanied by careful counselling regarding the risks to the fetus and consideration of invasive tests to detect fetal infection.

Herpes simplex virus
- Very rarely causes hepatitis but may do so in 3rd trimester or in the immunocompromized patient.
- Non-specific features—mucocutaneous stigmata may be absent and jaundice is not invariable.
- Prognosis for herpes simplex hepatitis is grave—mortality exceeding 90% even with treatment.

Gilbert's disease
- Affects 1–2% of population in Western world
- Mild flactuating jaundice
- May be more noticeable with dehydration, exhaustion, and poor calorie intake
- The increase in total bilirubin is a result of unconjugated hyperbilirubinaemia
- LFTs are normal and the patient is constitutionally well
- Does not pose any particular risks to pregnancy.

Autoimmune hepatitis
- Affects predominantly young women and leads to amenorrhoea so only earliest end of spectrum of disease encountered in obstetrics.
- Clinical features include rash, arthralgia, fever, malaise, anorexia, and weight loss and may often raise the possibility of SLE.
- Onset is insidious over weeks to months and often signs of chronic liver disease are present.
- LFTs are suggestive of hepatocellular injury but there may be associated derangements of hematological parameters (low platelets, low white cell count) and raised plasma globulins.
- Diagnosis is based on autoantibody studies showing the presence of anti smooth muscle antibodies and anti nuclear factor antibodies.

Cholecystitis
Decreased gallbladder motility and delayed emptying in pregnancy, lead to increase in gallbladder disease in pregnancy leading to asymptomatic gallstone disease in 3.5% of patients and acute cholecystitis with an incidence of 1 per 1000.

Clinical features
- Typically presents with severe epigastric and right upper quadrant pain often colicky in nature.
- Patient may be systemically unwell with fever, jaundice, nausea, and vomiting.
- There may be a previous history of gallstones.

Investigations
- LFTs may be deranged demonstrating a mixed hepatocellular/obstructive pattern. Serum amylase estimation should also be performed to exclude pancreatitis, as gallstones are a known predisposing factor for pancreatitis.

- An ultrasound scan of the upper abdomen may demonstrate gallstones and in cases of obstructive jaundice may show dilatation of the common bile duct. It may also exclude other causes of obstructive jaundice such as carcinoma of the head of pancreas or lymphadenopathy at the porta hepatis.

Management

- For acute cholecystitis, management involves supportive treatment
  - bed rest.
  - analgesia.
  - IV antibiotics (coamoxiclav or a combination of cephalosporin and metronidazole).
  - IV fluids.
  - period of resting the bowel. Nil by mouth.
  - if vomiting is a problem—nasogastric tube.
  - dietary advice of avoidance of fatty foods is essential for secondary prevention.
- Indications for surgical intervention
  - significant dilatation of the common bile duct suggestive of obstruction
  - empyema of gallbladder
  - recurrent attacks during pregnancy
  - pancreatitis.

Surgery during pregnancy carries a risk of preterm labour and hence risk need to be balanced and anticipated.

ⓘ **Diarrhoea in pregnancy**

Diarrhoea is loosely defined as passage of abnormally liquid or unformed stools at an increased frequency.

Normal physiological changes of pregnancy promote constipation, reported in up to one third of women during pregnancy. In contrast most cases of diarrhoea are not directly related to the pregnancy, but are due to the same disorders responsible for diarrhoea in non-pregnant women.

Causes

- Pregnancy related
  - Hormonal—increased prostaglandins eg; exacerbation of irritable bowel during pregnancy
- Not related to pregnancy
  - Infections (gastroenteritis)—bacterial, viral, protozoan
  - Medications—antibiotics, laxatives, prostaglandins
  - Inflammatory bowel disease
  - Malabsorption/maldigestion
  - Secondary to systemic infections e.g. listeriosis

More than 90% of cases of acute diarrhoea are caused by infectious agents.

Management

- History

Enquire about associated symptoms:

- onset of symptoms, any relation to recent intake of food in public restaurants and anyone else in the family or friends with similar symptoms (food poisoning).
- time interval—early onset (1–6 hr) suggests ingestion of preformed toxin (e.g. staph exotoxin)
- fever, vomiting, abdominal pain
- appearance of stool—bloody (shigella or campylobacter, amoebiasis and inflammatory bowel diseases), rice water (cholera)
- recent exposure to antibiotics—side effect or could be due to pseudo membranous colitis
- recent travel (travellers' diarrhoea).
- Examination
  - Assess for signs of dehydration and hypovolaemia
  - Any history and findings s/o preterm labour
  - Assessment of fetal heart.

Investigations

- FBC
- U&E
- stool examination
- culture and antibiotic sensitivity for bacteria
- analysis for ova and parasites
- faecal leucocytes—s/o intestinal inflammation
- stool assay for *Clostridium difficile* toxin—if there has been history of recent exposure to antibiotics

- flexible sigmoidoscopy—indicated in selected cases of prolonged diarrhoea not responding to usual conservative measures
- studies in pregnant patients have not been shown to be associated with any increased risk of complications.

Complications

In addition to the usual complications of diarrohea, pregnant patients are at increased risk of preterm labour, nosocomial spread to other pregnant patients (in a hospitalized patient), and to babies if strict aseptic precautions are not followed

Specific to organisms

- Campylobacter infection is associated with increased risk of spontaneous miscarriage, stillbirth, prematurity, and neonatal sepsis
- Salmonella typhi—risk of intrauterine transmission.

Treatment

Conservative management with fluid replacement is the mainstay of treatment

Low risk

- Dietary changes
- Fluid replacement—oral rehydration and/or IV fluids depending upon the severity of dehydration
- Increased fibre intake for irritable bowel syndrome (IBS)
- Fetal monitoring
- Medications
  - kaolin, pectin—adsorbents, no particular contraindication
  - in pregnancy but not shown to be effective in adults.
  - antibiotics—judicious use only if infectious aetiology is suspected, choice depending upon the aetiology.

Moderate risk

Loperamide & diphenoxylate (FDA drug risk category B*)

High risk

Bismuth subsalicylate (FDA drug risk category C*)

Routine use of antimotility drugs during pregnancy is not recommended.

(* For FDA drug risk category please refer to Pharmacotherapeutics in Obstetrics, Chapter 7.)

Obstetric complications

① Leakage of fluid

Leakage of fluid is the commonest presentation of rupture of fetal membranes (ROM) occurring at term (4–18%) or preterm (2%). This is the diagnosis that needs to be confirmed or refuted when the patient complaining of 'leakage of fluid' is assessed by the midwife or obstetrician.

Maternal risks

- Infection: the risk of systemic maternal infection antenatally at term is low, especially with appropriate management, although the rate of subclinical or histopathological chorioamnionitis is high.
- Higher risk of placental abruption.
- High incidence of obstetric intervention and associated risks if occurs prelabour (induction of labour, prolonged labour, increased risk of operative delivery).
- Postnatally the risks include endometritis and pelvic infection.
- In cases of preterm prelabour ROM (PPROM) there are also the psychosocial sequelae of a preterm baby possibly needing inpatient stay on the neonatal unit.

Fetal risks

The risks to the fetus increase significantly the lower the gestation at time of ROM.

- Infection: systemic sepsis, meningitis, and bronchopneumonia, especially where subclinical infection was the cause of underlying PPROM.
- With PPROM, prematurity and associated complications such as respiratory distress syndrome (RDS), necrotizing enterocolitis (NEC), bronchopulmonary dysplasia (BPD) and neurological problems.
- Fetal distress or fetal hypoxia due to cord compression, cord prolapse, abruption, infection, difficulties of delivering a premature infant.
- With extreme prematurity and marked reduction in amniotic fluid levels, there may be long term problems with pulmonary development and postural deformities.

Aetiology

Interaction of physical stresses with lack of resistance of fetal membranes.

- Before or during labour, cervical dilatation produces physical factors (lack of support), and biochemical factors (facilitated by infection of the chorioamnion) increase the probability of ROM.
- Weakness of the fetal membranes may be congenital or acquired (deficiency of vitamin C, smoking, infection within the amniotic cavity or over the part of the membranes overlying the cervical os).
- Infection may act by weakening the fetal membranes but also by an alternative mechanism involving the release of prostaglandins with resultant increase in uterine activity.

Diagnosis of prelabour rupture of membranes (PROM)

- Judicious assessment of patient history—timing of leakage and associated symptoms, amount of fluid lost (just dampness on underwear vs. soaked trouser/bed clothes), colour (clear/yellow, bloodstained, thick/dark green etc.), persistent loss after initial leak (need to use pads/change underwear). Any associated urinary symptoms.
- Diagnosis is based on visualization of either a pool of amniotic fluid in the posterior fornix or draining through the cervix at time of speculum examination. Confirmation of spontaneous ROM may be difficult if loss of fluid has subsided but may be helped by pressing on the uterine fundus, asking the patient to cough or perform the Valsalva manoeuvre with the speculum in situ. An alternative approach includes asking the patient to lie down for a couple of hours and repeating the speculum examination to see if a further pool of fluid has accumulated if initial exam was inconclusive.
- Diagnostic aids include nitrazine paper/sticks (orange) or red litmus paper which turn blue by amniotic fluid due to its alkaline pH but carry a false positive rate of 25% as alkalinization of the vagina may be caused by blood, semen, antiseptic, infected urine, *Trichomonas* infection, or bacterial vaginosis. Alternatively, when a sample of amniotic fluid is allowed to dry on a microscope slide, a fern pattern will be formed. Finally, the fetal fibronectin isoenzyme test may also provide confirmation of ROM.
- The role of ultrasound in diagnosis of SROM is controversial, as a loss of significant volume of fluid is required to be detectable on ultrasound. In the absence of demonstrable loss of fluid at early gestations, a 'wait and see' approach with repeated dry pads and a normal liquor volume on scan may provide supportive evidence that PPROM has not occurred.
- Differential diagnosis includes urinary stress incontinence, UTI and vaginal discharge. (Obtain MSU, genital swabs.)

Management

Best considered by grouping the pregnancies based on gestational age.

PROM at term (36 or more completed weeks)

- Confirm diagnosis and obtain HVS for culture (main concern is Group B Streptococcal colonization/infection).
- If cephalic presentation and otherwise low-risk pregnancy, expectant management for 24–48 hours for onset of labour (75–85% will labour in 24 hours and 90% by 48 hours).
- Patients asked to report bleeding, change in colour of liquor, fever, and reduced fetal movements.
- If labour does not supervene, then induction of labour by prostaglandin tablets or gel, oxytocin infusion or forewater ARM (if found to be present) should be recommended based on cervical assessment.
- Where there is suspicion of meconium staining of liquor, maternal fever, bleeding or other concerning features, safest policy is to proceed with induction of labour at the earliest opportunity.

Preterm PROM

Before 24 weeks

- Individualized management after full and frank discussion with parents depending on gestation and parental wishes.
- If continuation of pregnancy is chosen, expectant management as an outpatient after an initial period of hospitalization is being more commonly adopted.
- Baseline haematologicgal (FBC, CRP), microbiological (swabs, MSU) and ultrasound assessment of the fetus are performed.
- The mother is asked to monitor her own temperature, loss of fluid vaginally, other symptoms, restrict activity, and report any concerns.
- The patient can be reviewed on a weekly basis on an obstetric day unit, monitoring reaccumulation of fluid, haematological and microbiological parameters and fortnightly assessment for growth.
- The significance of the initial investment in counselling about the risks and guarded prognosis cannot be overstated.
- The pregnancy is continued until such point that the risks (for mother and/or baby) of continuing the pregnancy outweigh the benefits.

Between 24–34 weeks

- Confirmation of diagnosis and presentation.
- Baseline investigations: FBC, CRP, swabs and MSU. Ultrasound assessment of fetal wellbeing.
- Administration of betamethasone (24 mg IM in 2 doses over 12 hours apart) unless signs of overt sepsis.
- Commence patient on oral erythromycin 250 mgs qds for 10 days unless allergic to this antibiotic.
- If signs of preterm labour, a decision needs to be made on an individual basis regarding tocolysis to allow a window of opportunity to allow time for steroids to promote pulmonary maturity or transfer to unit with appropriate neonatal facilities. The decision will depend on gestation, other complicating issues such as bleeding or signs of infection, which would be contraindications to considering tocolysis.
- Where PPROM is followed by onset of preterm labour a decision regarding mode of delivery needs to be made. In general, if cephalic presentation then a vaginal delivery would be aimed for in the absence of fetal distress, history of placenta previa, previous classical CS or more than one previous lower segment CS. In cases of breech presentation or non-longitudinal lie, a CS would be recommended.
- Following PPROM, if labour does not supervene, than after a period of inpatient monitoring, the patient may be followed-up as an outpatient on a weekly basis on an obstetric day unit as above, until either 36–37 weeks of gestation are reached or maternal or fetal indications for delivery develop.

Between 34–36 weeks
- Similar to the 24–34 weeks gestation group, though the benefit of steroids is smaller and therefore use should be individualized.
- Antibiotics should be considered.
- Prolongation of pregnancy requires careful monitoring of maternal and fetal condition, using clinical (fetal movements), haematological, microbiological and biophysical (ultrasound) parameters of fetal wellbeing.
- The main benefit of prolongation of pregnancy at this stage is to improve the chances of a successful induction of labour and vaginal delivery.

☠ Bleeding in late pregnancy

Antepartum haemorrhage is bleeding from the genital tract in late pregnancy, occurring after viability (around 24 weeks gestation) and through till the intrapartum period. It affects 2–5% of pregnancies and can be a significant cause of fetal and maternal morbidity and mortality.

Main causes of antepartum haemorrhage

- Placenta previa: bleeding from a separation of an abnormally sited placenta.
- Abruption: bleeding from premature separation of a normally sited placenta.
- Bleeding from cervical or vaginal lesions (cervicitis, trauma, infections, vulvovaginal varicosities, genital tumours).
- Unknown cause.

Management

- Initial management depends on the cause and severity of bleeding and the gestational age of pregnancy.
- Maternal resuscitation if required: IV access with 2 wide bore cannulae, IV fluids, and blood if maternal condition warrants.
- Continuous monitoring and evaluation of fetal and maternal condition
- Reaching a diagnosis: history and examination—do not perform digital examination unless placenta previa excluded by US scan or examination is performed in theatre with set up for delivery by CS should a placenta previa be confirmed. Speculum examination after minimal bleeding and exclusion of PP may help identifying local causes of bleeding.
- Investigations: FBC, G&S serum or crossmatch blood according to need, coagulation screen where abruption is suspected, and Kleihauer test in Rhesus negative women. Ultrasound scan will help with placental localization.
- Continuing antenatal care: treat as high-risk the remainder of the pregnancy with serial monitoring of fetal growth and aim to deliver at term.

Placental abruption

Premature separation of a normally sited placenta occurs in 0.5–2.0% of pregnancies. The abruption may be revealed (blood tracks between the membranes and appears as vaginal bleeding), concealed (no vaginal bleeding), or mixed haemorrhage (vaginal bleeding but does not reflect the true extent of the abruption).

Risk factors

In most cases, no obvious cause. Potential causes include trauma and sudden uterine decompression such as with ROM in polyhydramnios. Other associations include maternal hypertension/pre-eclampsia, previous history of abruption (current or previous pregnancies), high parity, smoking, substance abuse (especially cocaine).

Maternal complications

Haemorrhage, hypovolaemic shock, DIC, renal failure, postpartum haemorrhage, maternal mortality and morbidity.

Fetal complications

Prematurity, growth restriction, intrapartum asphyxia, perinatal mortality.

Clinical features

Variable amount of vaginal bleeding associated with abdominal pain, uterine activity, and tender uterus. In large abruptions, there may be fetal distress or intrauterine fetal death (IUFD), haemodynamic collapse of the mother, along with increasing uterine fundal height/abdominal girth. The uterus feels 'woody' or 'hard', is irritable, and it may be difficult to palpate fetal parts. Backache may be an important symptom where the placenta is situated on the posterior uterine wall. Labour often supervenes in cases of significant abruptions.

Diagnosis

Clinical features are the most important clues as to the diagnosis. Large abruption may be visible on scan, the main role of the latter being to monitor growth and well being of the fetus in cases of conservative management.

Management

Depends on maternal and fetal condition, gestational age, severity of abruption, and presence of any other maternal complications.

- With large/severe abruption stabilization of maternal haemodynamic condition followed by delivery is needed. Maternal resuscitation and preparation for delivery need to occur concurrently.
- Mode of delivery will depend on whether the baby is alive, the prospects of achieving a vaginal delivery and the anticipated time-frame available before complications such DIC/fetal distress supervene.
- If in labour, it may be appropriate to perform an amniotomy to expedite this but where a decision to aim for a vaginal birth is made, continuous fetal monitoring is recommended.
- After a major abruption, careful postnatal monitoring is required with respect to maternal cardiovascular, renal and coagulation parameters.
- In cases of smaller abruptions especially at earlier gestations, conservative approach with initial hospitalization followed by close surveillance of fetal growth and welfare is appropriate with a view to delivery at term. If less than 34 weeks gestation, consider steroids.
- In Rhesus negative patients a Kleihauer test needs to be performed and appropriate amounts of anti-D immune globulin administered as required.

Placenta previa

The placenta is partially or completely inserted in the lower uterine segment. This complicates approximately 0.5% of pregnancies. Classification is based on site of placenta. Placenta previa (PP) is defined as minor (grade one and two) and major (grades three and four).

Grade one: placenta encroaching on lower segment but not reaching the os.
Grade two: placenta reaching the internal os.
Grade three: placenta covers the os but not centrally over it.
Grade four: placenta centrally across the os.

Majority of cases of minor degrees of PP identified in late 2nd and early 3rd trimester resolve by term.

Predisposing factors

Cause is unknown, but associated features include previous PP (5–10% recurrence), multiple pregnancy, multiparity, previous CS/uterine surgery, smoking and older mothers.

Clinical features

Unprovoked or postcoital painless vaginal bleeding. May be associated with malpresentation, unstable lie or an unengaged presenting part. A significant proportion are picked up on routine scanning. In the absence of routine scanning up to 15% may present in labour.

Diagnosis

Ultrasound scanning is the most commonly utilized diagnostic modality. The risk of false negative results is greater with a posterior PP as definition of the placental edge is harder in the absence of the contrast provided by the bladder when scanning an anterior placenta. MRI may be useful in inconclusive cases or examination in theatre at term is an alternative.

Management

This is determined in the acute phase by the mother's clinical condition, the fetal wellbeing, and the gestational age.
- Admit to hospital. The first bleed may be a small 'warning' bleed.
- Ensure mother is haemodynamically stable. (IV access, FBC, G&S serum/crossmatch as appropriate).
- Assess fetal wellbeing.
- If under 34 weeks gestation consider administration of steroids to promote pulmonary maturity.
- Where there is a major degree of placenta previa, especially with a history of antepartum bleeding, expectant management in hospital is warranted with repeated scans to assess placental edge (as lower segment form this may appear further from the internal os) and fetal growth/welfare (higher risk of IUGR with PP and recurrent bleeds).
- With minor degrees of PP examination in theatre, proceeding to amniotomy and induction of labour may be appropriate.
- If evidence of maternal or fetal compromise then maternal stabilization and delivery is indicated.
- If CS is warranted, senior obstetrician involvement is required, with crossmatched blood being available in theatre.
- In the presence of a history of previous CS and anterior PP, there is a significant risk of placenta acreta and need for Caesarean hysterectomy. At least 6 units of blood must be cross-matched. Senior obstetrician and anaesthetist should attend. Preoperative catheterization of internal iliac arteries, with the view to embolization to conserve the uterus or minimize bleeding, should be considered where facilities permit in cases where preoperative investigations suggest placenta arreata.

Antepartum haemorrhage and miscellaneous causes
Bleeding in pregnancy may arise from any part of the lower genital tract and occasionally from the lower urinary and gastrointestinal tract.

Bleeding from the lower genital tract
Causes
- Infection or inflammation of the cervix
- Cervical ectropion
- Cervical polyp
- Vulvovaginal trauma
- Vulval varicosities
- Cervical carcinoma.

Management
- Obtain history, especially of associated symptoms, including recent cervical cytology, pain, discharge, urinary, or bowel symptoms. Timing of recent intercourse in relation to vaginal bleeding.
- Clinical examination: inspection of vulva and a speculum examination when deemed to be safe (after placental localization by scan if required).
- Genital swabs may be appropriate to exclude infective causes of cervicitis.
- If the cervix looks abnormal then an experienced review to decide whether colposcopy is warranted should be considered.
- In Rhesus negative mothers a Kleihauer should be performed as missed diagnosis of maternal isoimmunization can have disastrous implications for future pregnancies.

☼ Leg pain and swelling in pregnancy

Definition
As a physiological response to a gravid uterus, bilateral/unilateral oedema/swelling is common. However pathological causes have to be ruled out.

Pathological causes
- Superficial thrombophlebitis
- Varicose veins
- Pre-eclampsia
- DVT
- Systemic disease i.e. heart failure, venous insufficiency, nephritic syndrome, liver failure, malabsorbsion, and malnutrition
- Drugs such as nifedipine
- Pelvic mass/malignancy
- Trauma/arthritis/compartment syndrome
- Necrotizing fasciitis
- Cellulitis
- Rupture Baker's Cyst.

Association
Thromboembolism is a major and leading cause of maternal mortality and morbidity. Untreated DVT may result in pulmonary embolism (PE) in up to 24% of patients with an associated mortality rate of 15 percent. Between 20–50% of cases occur antenatally. Bilateral, swollen, pitting legs are associated with systemic disease i.e. right-sided heart failure, hypoalbuminemia due to nephrotic syndrome, liver failure, malabsorbtion and malnutrition. Necrotizing fasciitis is associated with diabetes, trauma, and malignancy. Non-pitting oedema (lymph oedema) is related to infection and Milroy's syndrome.

Risk factors
The risk of DVT in pregnant women is 5–6 times higher than in non-pregnant women due to physiological hypercoagulable state in pregnancy, venous stasis, and bed rest. After operative deliveries the risk is increased to 10–20 fold and it increases even higher in those who had emergency Caesarean section.
   Other risk factors for DVT are:
- Age more than 40 years
- Parity above 5
- Oestrogen treatment to suppress lactation
- Sickle cell anaemia
- Obesity
- Blood group other than O
- Previous and family history of thromboembolism
- Prolonged immobility
- Malignancy
- Thrombophilia.

Presentation

- Varicose veins are common in pregnancy, occasionally associated with superficial thrombophlebitis.
- In DVT, calf swelling 2–3 centimetre greater than the other calf, calf tenderness, calf redness, increased warmth and distended veins, mild fever, pitting oedema, Homan's sign (calf pain in response to squeezing or stretching the Achilles tendon).
- Usually ilio-femoral (72% in pregnant vs. 9% in non-pregnant)— abdominal pain may be the only presenting sign.
- Left-sided DVTs in pregnancy (85% left vs. 15% right).
- 50% of patients who have classical DVT signs might not have DVT; therefore clinical assessment alone is not reliable in pregnancy.
- Bilateral pitting oedema, ↑JVP and hepatomegaly imply right-sided heart failure.
- Stiffness and knee swelling are related to Baker's cyst.
- Flu-like symptoms, ↑temperature, unilateral swelling, redness, and pain are related to cellulites.
- Headache, epigastria pain,↑BP and usually bilateral oedema is related to pre-eclampsia.
- Skin changes i.e. eczematous skin and ulcer is related to venous insufficiency.
- Drug history i.e. Ca channel blockers and vasodilators.
- Previous medical history i.e. systemic disease.
- Personal or family history of thromboembolisim.

Investigation

- Baseline assessment includes: full thrombophilia screening, FBC, urea, electrolytes, and LFT.
- Urine for protein.

If DVT is suspected

- The gold standard in diagnosis of DVT is venography, which has to be done with abdominal shielding. The estimation of radiation to the fetus is negligible.
- The non-invasive, highly effective investigation is real-time B-mode ultrasound and duplex Doppler. If the test is negative, and clinical suspicion is high, the test should be repeated after a few days.
- MRI and CT scan (little reported evidence of its use in pregnancy).
- D-Dimer (unreliable marker in pregnancy).
- If needed: ECG, CXR, Echo, ABG.

Management

- Anti-coagulants are the cornerstone of treatment of DVT.
- Heparin does not cross the placenta and therefore is the drug of choice. Oral anti-coagulant such as warfarin crosses the placenta and may cause embryopathy in the 1st trimester and intracerebral haemorrhage in the 2nd and 3rd trimesters.
- Heparin regimens include: continuous intravenous infusion of unfractionated heparin, subcutaneous injection of unfractionated heparin, or subcutaneous injections of low molecular weight heparin (LMWH).

- Subcutaneous LMWH is now considered an effective first line method.
- Recommended doses are: enoxaparin 1 mg/kg/BD, deltaparin 100 U/kg/BD up to a maximum of 18 000 U/24 hours, or tinzaparin 175 U/kg OD.
- Peak anti-Xa activity (3 hours post-injection) should be within the target therapeutic range. There is no need to repeat again if within range.
- Leg elevation and a graduated elastic compression stocking as well as mobilization. Women should be taught to self-inject until delivery.
- Treatment should be continued for at least 6 months if the DVT was above knee or 3 months if below knee.
- If DVT occurs early in the pregnancy, the dose of heparin could be reduced after 3 or 6 months according to location of DVT to prophylactic levels until 6 weeks postpartum.
- Warfarin can be used in the postpartum period. INR should be checked according to local protocols.
- During labour and delivery, the dose of heparin should be reduced to an intermediate dose roughly half-way between prophylactic and therapeutic doses.
- Epidural and spinal anaesthesia can be sited usually 12 hours after the last prophylactic dose and 24 hours after the last therapeutic dose to avoid the risk of epidural haematoma.
- Surgical embolectomy or thrombolytic therapy if DVT threatens leg viability.
- A caval filter may be required if recurrent venous thromboembolism (VTE), despite satisfactory anti-coagulation.

In systemic disease management is multidisciplinary
- In superficial thrombophlebitis—analgesia, compression stockings, leg elevation.
- In varicose veins—compression stockings.
- In necrotizing fasciitis remove all dead tissue and give benzylpenicillin.
- In compartment syndrome perform urgent fasciotomy.
- In Baker's cyst, aspiration is the treatment of choice.
- In cellulites treat with augmentin 375 mg/8h or erythromycin 500 mg/8h or phenoxymethylpenicillin 500 mg/4h po ± flucloxacillin 250 mg/6h po.

Further reading
1. Nelson-Piercy C (2002). Thrombo embolic disease. *Handbook of obstetric medicine*, 2nd edition. Martin Dunitz: London, 40–58.
2. Shehata HA, Nelson-Piercy C (2001). Medical diseases complicating pregnancy. *Anaes Inten Care Med*, **2**(6), 225–33.
3. Management of the High risk pregnancy obstetrics and gynaecology clinics of North America June 2004 volume 31 Michael O Grander.
4. Greer IA, ed. (1997) Thromboembolic disease in obstetrics and gynaecology. *Baillières Clin Obstet Gynaecol*, **11**, 431–45.
5. Report on Confidential Enquiry into Maternal Deaths in the United Kingdom 1994–96. London: HMSO, 1998.
6. Royal College of Obstetricians and Gynaecologists. Report of the RCOG Working Party on Prophylaxis against Thromboembolism in Gynaecology and Obstetrics. London: Chameleon Press, 1995.
7. Royal College of Obstetricians and Gynaecologists. Thromboembolic Disease in Pregnancy and the Puerperium: Acute Management. Guideline No. 28. London. April 2001.

⑦ Fainting episodes in pregnancy

Definition

Fainting is defined as transient loss of consciousness. A complaint of 'fainting' may not always imply actual loss of consciousness; some patients may mean no more than a feeling of unsteadiness or 'light-headedness'.

Associations

Convulsions, visual disturbances, vomiting, and sweating.

Causes

Vasomotor	Cardiac	Other causes
• Vasovagal attack	• Arryhythmia[3]	• Hyperventilation[1]
• Emotion[1]	• Aortic stenosis[3]	• Anxiety/panic attack[1]
• Fatigue[1]	• Hypertrophic cardiomyopathy[3]	• Eclampsia[3]
• Prolonged standing[1]	• Cyanotic attacks[3]	• Epilepsy[2]
• Chronic illness[1]	• Ischaemic heart disease[3]	• Hypoglycaemia[3]
• Haemorrhage (ectopic, placental abruption, post-partum)[3] internal bleeding[4]		• Diabetic ketoacidosis[3]
• Severe pain[2]		• Massive pulmonary embolism
• Postural hypotension[2]		• Electrolyte Imbalance[1]
• Supine hypotension[2]		• Transient ischaemic attack (TIA)[2]
• Carotid-sinus syncope[2]		• Carbon monoxide poisoning[3]

Diagnostic steps

Take a proper history from the patient. A witness is important for proper diagnosis. Secure airway, breathing, and circulation. It is a serious emergency if haemorrhage or massive pulmonary embolism led to the fainting attack. Loss of consciousness and duration of the attack is <2 minutes in vasovagal syncope. It is more in SVT or other arrhythmia and is seconds in Stokes–Adams attacks. A fall, injury, and biting tongue may indicate epilepsy. Urinary incontinence during and post attack is rare in vasovagal syncope but common in epilepsy or TIA. Presence of hypertension, oedema, and proteinuria indicate ecclampsia. Warning symptoms may suggest vasovagal syncope, epilepsy or postural hypotension. Confusion or sleepiness may occur in epilepsy. Other associated factors such as palpitation, chest pain and breathlessness may indicate cardiac disease. Drug history such as insulin therapy, alcohol, or B-blockers may cause fainting.

Vital signs measurement, cardiovascular assessment and neurological examination are essential. BP measurement in supine and standing positions, respiratory rate and temperature are essential.

Investigations

- FBC
- U&Es
- Urine dipstick for proteins and ketones
- Plasma glucose
- TFT in arrhythmia
- Pulse oximetry
- ECG, identify the rate, QRS width, configuration of p wave to differentiate SVT/AF/VT/heart block
- Echo for LV function and to exclude structural abnormality
- Blood culture
- MSU and CXR if infection is suspected
- Arterial blood gas if hypoxic
- EEG, sleep EEG
- CT and/or MRI if necessary.

Management

- In heamodynamically unstable patient—manage with ABC
- Involve relevant specialities accordingly (multi-disciplinary management).

Vasomotor

Postural and supine hypotension are relieved by assuming lateral position to reduce pressure of the gravid uterus on the inferior vena cava.

Cardiac arrhythmia

- Identify the underlying rhythm and treat accordingly.
- Give oxygen and get IV access.
- In SVT try vagotonic manoeuvres (carotid sinus massage or Valsalva manouvre). If unsuccessful, treat with adenosine. Fetal monitoring should be preformed at the time as fetal bradycardia has been reported.
- Frequent symptomatic episodes of SVT need treatment with β-blockers, calcium channel blockers, digoxin and quinidine.
- Flecainide has been used for treatment of SVT in Wolff–Parkinson–White syndrome in pregnancy.
- Episodes of VT can be due to cathecolamine sensitivity and are triggered by stress or exertion and suppressed with β-blockers.
- Direct current cardioversion is indicated for maternal and fetal hemodynamic instability.
- Amiodarone should be avoided if possible but can be used if benefit outweighs the risks of neonatal thyroid dysfunction.
- Anti-coagulation requirements depend on the presence of additional risk factors, including LV function impairment identified by echocardiography.
- Low dose aspirin 75 mg could be used when no additional risk factors are identified.

Diabetic ketoacidosis

- Calculate the fluid requirement (maintenance of 150 ml/kg normal saline).
- Add 20 mmol KCl to the fluid except the first litre if not oliguric or K >6.
- Replace the fluid aggressively with normal saline over 24 hours. 1 L stat, followed by 1 L over next hour, then 1 L over 2 hours, then 4 hours, then 6 hours.
- Sliding scale for insulin, if BM >20 mmol/L.
- Aim for blood glucose 4–8 mmol/L for the first 24 hours, maintain this with 5% dextrose infusion.
- Monitor the patient closely for vital signs.
- Transfer patient to HDU or ITU if required.
- Treat suspected infection with antibiotic.

Hypoglycaemia

- A plasma blood glucose <2.2 mmol/L is associated with a severe attack and coma occurs with levels <1.5 mmol/L.
- If conscious treat with oral sugar and 50 g of oral glucose.
- If unconscious, 25 or 50 g glucose IV or 50–100 ml of 50% dextrose IV fast followed by 0.9% saline flush. Or glucagons 0.5 to 1mg S/C or IM if IV access impossible. Repeat after 20 min following with carbohydrate. Do not give further IV bolus of glucose until repeat blood sugar is performed.
- If not conscious after 10 min consider another cause, e.g. head injury.
- Recurrent hypoglycemia may indicate diabetic nephropathy.

References

1. Shotan A, et al. (1997). Incidence of arrhythmias in normal pregnancy and relation to palpitations, dizziness, and syncope. Am J Cardiol, 79(8), 1061–4.
2. Arici A, Copel JA (2004). Endocrinology of pregnancy. Obstetrics and Gynecology Clinics of North America, **31**(4), 907–35.
3. Nelson-Piercy C (2002). Respiratory disease. In: Nelson-Piercy C (ed.). Handbook of obstetric medicine, 2nd edition. London: Martin Dunitz, 59–81.
4. Kniseley RM (1995). Acute internal bleeding as a cause of syncope. Am Fam Physician, **52**(5), 1278.

⑦ Pyrexia in pregnancy

Fever is both a symptom and a sign which should be taken seriously during antepartum, intrapartum, and postpartum periods. Although it is often due to common bacterial and viral infections, other rare but potentially fatal causes like chorioamnionitis, deep vein thrombosis (DVT) and sub-acute bacterial endocarditis (SABE) need to be excluded during pregnancy. The risks to the fetus may be three fold: vertical transmission of infections leading to congenital infection, teratogenicity, or fetal death; direct effect of hyperpyrexia on developing fetal brain; and the possibility of preterm labour. The fetus may also be affected due to the investigations to diagnose, and the treatment of, the underlying cause of pyrexia.

It may be useful to consider the causes of pyrexia during antepartum, intrapartum, and postpartum periods separately.

Causes—antepartum period
Infections
- Organ specific
  - Urinary tract (cystitis, pyelonephritis)
  - Respiratory tract (tracheo-bronchitis, basal pneumonia, tuberculosis)
  - Uterine—chorioamnionitis
  - Gastrointestinal—hepatitis, pancreatitis, enteritis, appendicitis
  - Cardiac—sub-acute bacterial endocarditis (SABE)
  - Neurological—meningitis, encephalitis
- Systemic
  - Viral (including rubella, varicella, cytomegalovirus, herpes simplex infections)
  - Bacterial—septicaemia
  - Protozoal—toxoplasmosis, malaria, amoebiasis.

Dehydration
Severe hyperemesis gravidarum.

Adnexal accidents
- Torsion, haemorrhage into or rupture of ovarian cysts
- Torsion of pedunculated fibroid
- Red degeneration of fibroids.

Endocrine/metabolic
Diabetic ketoacidosis, phaeochromocytoma, hyperthyroidism.

Thrombosis
DVT, pulmonary embolism.

Malignancies
Lymphomas, leukaemias.

Pyrexia of unknown origin (PUO)

Others
Sickle cell crisis.

Causes—intrapartum period

- Chorioamnionitis: any of the antepartum causes can result in pyrexia during labour. It is important to exclude chorioamnionitis. If untreated, this can result in serious consequences to the mother (septicaemia, DIC, and death) and to the fetus (fetal compromise and death; neonatal sepsis including encephalitis and possible long term neurological sequelae). The following risk factors should be considered:
  - prolonged rupture of membranes
  - prolonged labour, especially with repeated vaginal examinations
  - presence of vaginal discharge.
- Dehydration: due to prolonged labour/diabetic keto-acidosis.

Causes—postpartum period

Puerperal sepsis

This is the commonest cause of pyrexia following delivery. It is defined as any fever >38°C on 2 or more occasions, excluding the first 24 hours and up to 14 days of delivery or miscarriage. Causes are as follows:
- 90% are due to genital tract (endometritis, pelvic abscess) and urinary tract (cystitis, pyelonephritis) infections.
- Breast engorgement/acute mastitis/breast abscess.
- Respiratory tract infections including basal pneumonia.
- DVT/septic thrombophlebitis secondary to pelvic infection.
- Wound infection—caesarean section, episiotomy, perineal tears.

Other causes

Any systemic or organ specific infections of the antepartum period may also occur during the postpartum period.

Associated clinical features

- Malaise, lethargy, myalgia, arthralgia, rash—systemic viral infections
- Chills and rigors—UTI, malaria
- Abdominal pain, nausea, vomiting, alteration in bowel habits—acute gastroenteritis, acute appendicitis
- Jaundice, loss of appetite, anorexia—hepatitis, pancreatitis
- Dysuria, haematuria, pyuria, loin to groin pain—UTI
- Ketone breath, 'Cheyene–Stokes' breathing—diabetic ketoacidosis
- Calf pain, swelling, redness—DVT
- Abdominal pain, vaginal discharge—chorioamnionitis, endometritis
- Pain, redness or engorgement of breasts, nipple discharge— acute mastitis, breast abscess
- Swinging temperatures, deterioration of clinical condition—pelvic abscess, septic thrombophlebitis
- Cough with sputum, haemoptysis—respiratory tract infections
- Onset of hypothermia and hypotension in a patient who has be previously pyrexial may indicate septicaemia.

Examination

A detailed and systematic clinical examination should be performed to identify the cause of pyrexia. The following approach may be useful:

General examiation
- Level of consciousness, degree of pyrexia, hydration
- Rash
- Jaundice, cyanosis.

Head and neck
- Cervical lymphadenopathy
- Neck stiffness
- Thyroid gland, toxic nodular goiter.

Chest
- Cardiovascular system: vital signs/clubbing/changing murmurs
- Respiratory system: air entry, breath sounds, added sounds, evidence of consolidation
- Breasts: engorgement, redness, nipple discharge.

Abdominal examination
- Abdominal wall: tenderness, guarding, rigidity, rebound tenderness (signs of peritoneal irritation).
- Hepatic/epigastric tenderness (pancreatitis).
- Tenderness over McBurney's Point is **not** a reliable sign to diagnose acute appendicitis in pregnancy due to the upward displacement of the caecum by the gravid uterus. Tenderness may be elicited right up to the right hypochondrium.
- Palpable liver (hepatitis), spleen (SABE, malaria).
- Iliac fossae—adnexal masses, tenderness.
- Uterus—tenderness (chorioamnionitis), masses (red degeneration of fibroids).

Wounds
Abdominal, perineal, genital tract for evidence of infection.

Calves
- Swelling, tenderness, red or blue discoloration
- Homan's sign and Moses's sign are best avoided to prevent the possible dislodgement of the clot.

Spine
Infection at the site of spinal and epidural anaesthesia.

Investigations

It is important to perform appropriate investigations based on the history and clinical examination findings to confirm the diagnosis and to monitor the response to treatment.
- FBC
- Blood urea and serum electrolytes
- LFTs
- MSU
- C-Reactive protein (CRP)
- Swabs—high vaginal/endocervical swabs/wound/nipple

- Blood cultures (chorioamnionitis, septicaemia)
- CXR (with abdominal shield prior to delivery)
- Sputum for microscopy and culture
- Urine for ketones
- Blood gases (diabetic ketoacidosis, septicaemia)
- Abdominal ultrasound—to assist in the diagnosis of pelvic abcess, pyometra
- Doppler ultrasound scan—calf vein thrombosis, iliofemoral vein thrombosis. If pulmonary embolism is suspected, a ventilation/perfusion scan (V/Q scan) should be performed
- Blood for malarial parasites—if suspected
- Lumbar puncture—if meningitis or encephalitis is suspected.

Management

This depends on the cause and may require a 'multi-disciplinary approach' in some situations (e.g. DVT, malignancies, diabetic keto-acidosis, appendicitis). Anti-pyretics may be indicated to control pyrexia while specific treatment is essential to eradicate the underlying cause.

Infections
- Antibiotics—intravenously in severe cases
- Antivirals
- Anti-protozoal—for malaria, toxoplasmosis, amoebiasis.

Dehydration
Intravenous fluids, insulin and bicarbonate infusion in diabetic ketoacidosis.

Chorioamnionitis
- Induction of labour
- Intravenous broad spectrum antibiotics once the diagnosis is made. This should be continued during labour and in the immediate postpartum period.

Endometritis
Broad spectrum antibiotics, monitoring of involution and exclusion of retained products of conception.

Deep vein thrombosis
Anticoagulants, TED stocking, involvement of a haematologist.

Surgical management
Acute appendicitis, adnexal accidents and pelvic or breast abscess may warrant surgical intervention.

Fetal monitoring
Toxoplasmosis, rubella, cytomegalovirus, herpes simplex virus, and syphilitic infections may be transmitted transplacentally, leading to fetal malformation or intrauterine growth restriction. If the mother is not immune to these infections and if one of these infections is suspected (or confirmed), she should be counselled regarding the possible detrimental effects and the plan of management.

A scan may be arranged after 5 weeks of infection to identify any structural defects. Serial ultrasound scans may be required to identify intrauterine growth restriction.

Conclusion

Pyrexia during pregnancy, labour, and puerperium needs to be investigated and treated appropriately. Although urinary tract infections are one of the commonest causes of pyrexia in pregnancy, other more potentially serious causes need to be excluded. A systematic approach to history taking and examination may help to decide on the most appropriate investigations to help in the diagnosis. The effects of pyrexia as well its underlying cause on the fetus should be recognized.

☼ Painful uterine contractions

Introduction

Pain arising from any smooth muscle organ may be due to ischaemia, irritation, or injury. It is important to distinguish physiological causes of painful uterine contractions (during labour and 'after pains' following delivery) from pathological uterine contractions. As a general rule, physiological contractions are intermittent whereas pathological contractions are often continuous or sustained. They may also be associated with other clinical features like vaginal bleeding, fever, and changes in fetal heart trace.

It may be useful to consider the pathological causes of painful uterine contractions during the first half of pregnancy, second half of pregnancy, during labour, and in the immediate puerperium separately.

First half of pregnancy

- Threatened miscarriage—mild pain and small amount of bleeding
- Inevitable and incomplete miscarriage—more severe pain/bleeding
- Septic miscarriage—continuous pain/fever/feeling unwell
- Pregnancy in a uterine horn/cornual pregnancy—colicky pain that may present with signs of intra-abdominal bleeding.

Second half of pregnancy

- Late miscarriage
- Preterm labour—idiopathic, uterine over-distension (multiple pregnancy, polyhydraminos, fibroids)
- Uterine irritability (abruption, chorioamnionitis, pyelonephritis and following procedures like amniocentesis or external cephalic version).

During labour

- Uterine hyperstimulation (injudicious use of oxytocin)
- Placental abruption
- Uterine scar dehiscence/rupture
- Intrapartum infections (chorioamnionitis, pyelonephritis).

After delivery

- Retained products of conception
- Acute inversion of the uterus.

Clinical approach

A detailed antenatal history should be taken and risk factors, if present, should be noted (e.g. augmentation of labour with oxytocin, multiple pregnancy, previous history of abruption, pre-eclampsia). It may be useful to identify the nature of pain and associated factors as follows:

Nature of pain

- Intermittent, progressive pain—preterm labour, late miscarriage
- Colicky abdominal pain—inevitable or incomplete miscarriage, cornual ectopic pregnancy, retained products after delivery

- Continuous sharp pain/breakthrough pain in between contractions—placental abruption, uterine scar dehiscence, or rupture
- Constant dull ache—uterine irritation (chorioamnionitis, septic miscarriage, pyelonephritis, red degeneration of a fibroid).

Associated features
- Vaginal bleeding—miscarriage, preterm labour, abruption, scar dehiscence or rupture, retained products of conception
- Vaginal discharge—septic miscarriage, chorioamnionitis
- Fever—pyelonephritis (with loin to groin pain, dysuria, haematuria, pyuria), chorioamnionitis, septic miscarriage.

Signs
General examination
- Shock/collapse—rupture of cornual pregnancy, placental abruption, uterine rupture, uterine inversion, severe sepsis, or severe haemorrhage
- Pallor
- Raised temperature—infection, irritation, inflammation
- Tachycardia/hypotension—severe bleeding, sepsis
- Bradycardia/hypotension—uterine inversion.

Abdominal examination
- Symphysio-fundal height—multiple pregnancy, polyhydraminos (tense abdomen, shiny skin)
- Uterine tenderness—placental abruption, chorioamnionitis, red degeneration of fibroid
- Frequency and duration of contractions
- Abdominal wall guarding, rigidity, tenderness or rebound tenderness—peritoneal irritation (chorioamnionitis, uterine rupture). Uterine 'scar tenderness' is a non-specific sign
- Fluid thrill—polyhydraminos
- Renal angle tenderness—pyelonephritis
- Epigastric/hypochondrial tenderness (if abruption is a part of pre-eclamptic process).

Cardiotocograph (CTG)
- Baseline fetal heart rate
  - *Tachycardia* (infections, fetal compromise, uterine rupture)
  - *Bradycardia* (severe fetal compromise).
- Baseline variability: *poor variability* (0–5) fetal compromise—for >90 min.
- Decelerations: *late or prolonged decelerations are* ominous suggestive of acute fetal compromise secondary to placental abruption or scar rupture.
- Changes in uterine contractions ('TOCO'):
  - *Increased frequency* (>6/10 min)—uterine hyperstimulation/ irritability
  - *Increased baseline tone*—placental abruption, impending uterine rupture. After rupture, the contractions may not be recordable.

Examination of the lower genital tract
• To confirm vaginal bleeding (abruption, miscarriage, uterine rupture) or vaginal discharge or rupture of membranes (chorioamnionitis)
• To assess any cervical change (miscarriage/preterm labour)
• To take high vaginal swabs or to diagnose and correct uterine inversion.

Investigations (depending on the cause)
• FBC
• Blood urea and serum electrolytes
• CRP—infection/inflammation
• MSU for microscopy, culture and sensitivity—pyelonephritis
• Blood cultures—for chorioamnionitis, severe pyelonephritis
• Kleihauer test—suspected abruption (possible feto-maternal haemorrhage)
• Clotting profile—abruption, severe sepsis
• Ultrasound scan—not very useful in an acute clinical situation. It may be helpful in the diagnosis of multiple pregnancy, polyhydraminos, retained products, miscarriage, and cornual pregnancy. Fetal viability could be determined by ultrasound scan that may influence clinical decisions regarding further management.

Management
Depends on the cause of painful uterine contractions and may necessitate a multi-disciplinary approach involving anaesthetists (fluid and pain management), haematologists (severe haemorrhage), microbiologists (sepsis) and neonatologists.

Miscarriage/retained products of conception	**Evacuation of retained products (ERPC)**
Chorioamnionitis/ pyelonephritis/ septicaemia	**IV antibiotics/IV fluids, pain relief, multi-organ support** If fetus in utero consider delivering by induction or CS
Preterm labour	**Tocolytics** (if indicated) Betamethasone Plan for transfer or mode of delivery if no response to tocolytics
Uterine hyperstimulation	**Stop oxytocin infusion, improve uterine perfusion** (IV fluids, left lateral position) Consider—**acute tocolysis** (terbutaline 0.25 mg SC)
Placental abruption	**Resuscitate, consider delivery if likely to cause fetal compromise** (abnormal ctg, uterine irritability) or maternal compromise (haemodynamic disturbance)
Uterine rupture/cornual ectopic pregnancy	**Emergency laparotomy**
Uterine inversion	**Replacement of uterine fundus under anaesthetic if immediate manual replacement was not undertaken** Atropine if in neurogenic shock

Key points

- Differentiate physiological from pathological causes of painful uterine contractions.
- Take relevant history, identify risk factors, perform detailed clinical examination and appropriate investigations to diagnose the possible cause as well as complications.
- Consider multi-disciplinary approach whenever necessary.
- Assess maternal and fetal condition prior to clinical decision making.
- If appropriate, consider early:
  - anti-D (if Rhesus negative)
  - antenatal corticosteroids
  - in-utero transfer.

⑦ Abnormal vaginal discharge in pregnancy

This is a common complaint among pregnant women. The symptoms are often managed empirically, leading to inaccurate diagnosis and ineffective management.

Normal vaginal discharge is produced daily at the rate of 1–4 ml/day. It is typically white/clear and odourless. The discharge consists of vaginal transudate, epithelial cells, cervical mucus, and normal vaginal flora. The most common vaginal commensal is *Lactobacillus acidophilus*.

Causes

- Physiological: normal vaginal discharge can be in excessive amounts in some women.
- Infective: candidiasis, bacterial vaginosis, chlamydia, gonorrhoea, trichomoniasis
- Rare: malignancy, foreign body, douches.

Management

History

- *Duration of symptoms*
  - recent
  - longstanding
  - intermittent.
- *Amount*
  - scanty
  - copious.
- *Colour*
  - greenish
  - white mucusy
  - blood stained
  - clear watery.
- *Itching*
  - severe itching
  - no itching.
- *Change in nature:* becoming bloodstained from a clear or white mucusy discharge
- *Odour*
  - hygienic problem
  - odourless
  - fishy smell
  - uriniferous odour.

Examination

- Local: look for signs of itching, erythema, oedema, fissures on the vulval skin.
- Speculum
  - amount and nature of discharge
  - appearance of cervix
  - soreness on examination

Common causes of vaginal discharge in pregnancy

Likely cause	Appearance	pH	Microscopy	When to treat	Treatment
Normal	Milky, white/clear, odourless,		Lactobacilli	Reassure	
Candidiasis	White, adherent (curd like), sore on examination	4.0–4.5	Hyphae present	Treat symptomatic women	Clotrimazole pessary 500 mg stat. Use cream for 7–14 days to treat vulvitis
Bacterial vaginosis	Clear/thin, homogenous, fishy odour	>4.5	Reduced lactobacilli, clue cells	Associated with preterm labour. Treat if previous history of preterm labour with infective etiology	Clindamycin 2%, 1 applicator full once daily × 7 days. Metronidazole 400 mg twice daily × 7 days
Chlamydia	Mucopurulent	Variable	Increased polymorphs. Gram's stain may show lactobacilli	Treat	Erythromycin 500 mg BD × 14 days
Gonorrhoea	Mucopurulent	Variable	As above. Gram negative intracellular diplococci on culture	Treat	Inj. Ceftriaxone 250 mg IM stat
Group B Streptococcus	Variable	Variable	Gram staining shows streptococci	Treat if symptomatic otherwise needs antibiotic prophylaxis in labour	Treat as per sensitivity. Usually sensitive to penicillin
Trichomoniasis	Grayish green, frothy discharge, *strawberry punctuation* of cervix	>4.9	Motile protozoa seen	Treat	Metronidazole 200 mg three times daily for 7 days

- any obvious odour
- Take high vaginal swab (HVS) and endocervical swabs for chlamydia and gonorrhoea.

Digital vaginal examination is not always necessary. It may be done when the cervix cannot be clearly seen and there is a chance the patient could be in labour.

Treatment

General

Local hygiene

- Keep area dry
- avoid perfumed detergents locally if sore
- avoid douches.

Specific

See table.

Differential diagnosis

- Ruptured membranes—clear, watery fluid
- Urinary incontinence—episodic, clear fluid, uriniferous odour.

⚠ Frequency of micturition and acute retention of urine

The anatomical and physiological changes in pregnancy are associated with significant changes in the functions of the upper and lower urinary tract. The changes are so extensive that non-pregnant norms are inappropriate for pregnant patients. Awareness of this is essential to detect early signs of urinary tract dysfunction to prevent damage that may have long term effects.

Antenatal problems

Frequency of micturition

Frequency is defined as greater than 7 daytime voids and 1 night-time void. One of the earliest symptoms of pregnancy is urinary frequency and this can be even be noticed before the first missed period. Urinary frequency in pregnancy is secondary to the hyperdynamic circulation and increased urine production by the kidneys.

Urinary frequency increases as pregnancy progresses. Pressure from the enlarging uterus or the presenting part may directly irritate the trigone and cause urinary frequency. Frequency is usually more common in nulliparous than multiparous mothers. Black nulliparous women are more prone to have increased frequency compared to White nulliparous and Black parous women are more prone to increased nocturia compared to White parous women.

The majority of women accept increased urinary frequency and nocturia as a normal part of pregnancy and will put up with it. Only a few (less than 4%) are actually distressed.

Urinary tract infections can present with increased urinary frequency, dysuria, nocturia, and urgency. Diagnosis on the basis of symptoms is difficult as these symptoms are considered as a normal part of pregnancy. Therefore diagnosis must be based on urine testing or laboratory evidence. Presence of leucocytes, proteins, and nitrites on dipstick examination suggests the possibility of urinary tract infection and the need to send a mid-stream sample of urine (MSU) for culture and antibiotic sensitivity test (ABST). A colony count of more than 100 000 bacteria per ml of urine is regarded as infection although a count of as low as 20 000 may represent acute infection in pregnancy. Urinary white cell count also increases in pregnancy. *E. coli* is the common infective agent and *Proteus*, *Klebsiella* and *Enterobacter* account for most of the remainder.

Management of antenatal urinary frequency

- Reassurance: patients need advice and reassurance (after excluding a urinary tract infection) that increased urinary frequency is part of the normal physiological changes of pregnancy, it is benign in nature and will gradually resolve after pregnancy.
- Urine testing: in pregnancy, 5% of women will have asymptomatic bacteriuria, 30% of whom will develop a symptomatic infection if untreated. Urinary infection increases the risk of complications in

pregnancy such as preterm labour and fetal growth restriction. Therefore a MSU sample should be taken at the booking to exclude infection if urinary screening suggests infection. Additional screening (usually monthly) for infection is indicated in women with past history of urinary tract infections and/or renal disorders. Antimicrobials should be based on the culture and sensitivity report and continued for at least 7–10 days for initial infections and 21 days for recurrences.

Retention of urine

Urinary retention in pregnancy usually presents as an acute episode though its development may have been slow over several days or weeks. During the antenatal period the commonest time for its development is during the 1st trimester.

The classic cause of retention during the 1st trimester is incarceration of the retroverted uterus. The mechanism of urinary obstruction has traditionally thought to be due to pressure on the bladder neck from the uterus but as there is often no difficulty in passing a urinary catheter the exact mechanism of the blockage remains unclear.

Clinical presentation is usually the inability to pass urine in association with pelvic pain. The bladder may or may not be palpable abdominally. Inspection of fluid charts may be falsely reassuring as the patient may be in chronic urinary retention with incomplete bladder emptying. It is therefore important to include assessment of post-void urinary residual volume estimation using either ultrasound estimation or passage of a urinary catheter.

Management of antenatal urinary retention

Once urinary retention has been diagnosed immediate passage of a urinary catheter will result in relief of pain. Measurement of the volume of urine within the bladder should be performed as sustained volumes over 800 ml may be associated with longer term urinary dysfunction (see postpartum, below). Urine should also be tested for urinary tract infection which is commonly found in association with urinary stasis.

The catheter should be left in situ and when the patient is comfortable a gentle vaginal examination should be performed to assess the degree of uterine incarceration. Occasionally the patient may be relieved of the incarceration by spending periods lying prone or on all fours in a 'knee–chest' position. The catheter should remain in until the uterus remains reliably out of the pelvis. The patient should be warned that this may take several weeks.

Once the catheter is removed the patient should be observed for several hours to assess voided volumes and estimated urinary residuals using ultrasound. If the urinary residual is reliably less than 100 ml the patient may be discharged. Several days later further urinary residual estimation should be performed to ensure chronic retention does not ensue.

Intrapartum problems

Retention of urine

During labour, retention of urine may be pathophysiological or iatrogenic. Part of the normal assessment of the healthy woman in labour should include recording of urine output. The commonest causes of low urine volumes are dehydration and retention of urine. Due to the compressive effects of the descending fetal head the likelihood of urinary retention increases as labour progresses. If the patient is unable to void then the presence of obstruction can be distinguished by clinical inspection and palpation and confirmed by ultrasound assessment of urinary residual or with the use of intermittent catheterization.

Epidural analgesia is associated with loss of bladder sensation and though intermittent catheterization is an acceptable way of managing urine flow during the labour of a woman who wishes to remain mobile and has an epidural, it is important that attention is paid to the bladder, ensuring it is emptied at least every 2 hours. In the woman who is less mobile with an epidural it may be appropriate to insert an indwelling catheter.

All women who have spinal anaesthesia for instrumental deliveries or caesarean section should have an indwelling catheter inserted until sensation is fully restored.

Management of intrapartum urinary retention

This should be with the use of an indwelling urinary catheter which should remain in situ until the patient is mobile following delivery or until the epidural is no longer functioning.

Puerperium

Frequency of micturition

Normal pregnancy is associated with an increase in extracellular fluid and puerperal diuresis is a reversal of this process. Increased urinary frequency between the 2nd and 5th postpartum day is primarily due to this diuresis. Thereafter urinary frequency gradually resolves although the presence of enlarged uterus could to some extent continue to give rise to frequency and urgency. Factors during labour such as haemorrhage or pre-eclampsia can influence the normal puerperal diuresis and frequency. Epidural analgesia in labour can alter bladder sensation and hence the frequency of micturition.

Retention of urine

One of the commonest causes of long-term bladder damage is that caused by an episode of acute urinary retention during the immediate postpartum period. Overdistension may be as a consequence of either perineal trauma producing urethral oedema or as a result of reduced bladder sensation following regional analgesia or anaesthesia.

The damage that can result from overdistension with sustained volumes greater than 800 ml includes acute pain, and in severe cases bladder rupture and mucosal haemorrhage. If the retention goes unrecognized for long periods of time there may be damage to the neural network within the bladder. This may result in reduced bladder sensation and detrusor muscle hypocontractility. If it goes unrecognized it can lead to longstanding voiding difficulties and its accompanying chronic problems such as infection and renal damage.

Management of postpartum urinary retention

It is particularly important that action is taken immediately if a woman is found postnatally to be suspected of going into urinary retention. The timely insertion of a urinary catheter may relieve the pain but if follow-up action is not taken over the next 2–4 hours long-term damage may result as the bladder refills. It is therefore important to measure the urine volume upon catheterization and to leave an indwelling catheter for 24 hours if the volume is over 800 ml. When the catheter is removed, post-void urinary residual volumes should be estimated after every void until they are reliably less than 100 ml.

In some cases where there has been extreme or late recognition of bladder overdistention the bladder damage may not show signs of recovery in the short term. This may mean there has been permanent damage that will need long-term methods of ensuring complete bladder emptying such as intermittent clean self-catheterization or long-term indwelling catheter. All cases will need close multidisciplinary follow-up in combination with continence specialists and specialist physiotherapists. Often it is possible to significantly improve, and in some cases cure, voiding dysfunction in women who have had severe bladder damage from acute postpartum urinary retention.

With the correct patient care pathways and guidelines in place for the management of urinary tract function during pregnancy, cases of severe bladder damage should be avoided.

Concerns for the fetus and surveillance

Amarnath Bhide, Padma Vankayalapati, and Nicholas Ngeh

ⓘ Absent fetal movements

Normal pattern of fetal movements

Although fetal limb and body movements are visible on ultrasound from the 1st trimester, maternal perception starts only after 16–20 weeks of gestation. Typically the fetus demonstrates sleep–wake cycles every 40 minutes, where a period of active movements alternate with a period of quiescence. Towards the end of pregnancy the pattern of fetal movements often changes. Relative reduction in the available space and engagement of the head are some of the factors responsible for this change.

Significance of absent fetal movements

It was historically noted that in pregnancies complicated by intrauterine fetal death, fetal movements typically ceased 12–24 hours prior to disappearance of fetal heart activity. This sign was called the movement alarm signal (MAS). It was theorized that a hypoxic fetus saved energy by reducing fetal activity.

Application of this information to the general low-risk obstetric population, however, did not show benefit. In fact, there was a trend towards worse fetal outcome when interventions were carried out prompted by fetal movement reduction. Loss or a reduction of fetal movements generates considerable parental anxiety. Absence or reduction of fetal movements is a useful sign for monitoring pregnancies where ongoing fetal hypoxia is a likely possibility.

Clinical applications
- Placental insufficiency
- Post-term pregnancy
- Medical complications such as diabetes in pregnancy or obstetric cholestasis
- Fetal anaemia such as Rhesus disease
- Fetal cardiac failure
- Fetal hypoxia due to any cause.

Evaluation of the patient

Evaluation is aimed at establishing the risk status of the pregnancy.

History—present and past
- The history of reduction or loss of fetal movements should be explored in greater detail. The previous pattern should be established.
- Essentially, the history forms a part of risk assessment.
- Placental insufficiency is more common in the first pregnancy. It is extremely uncommon in subsequent pregnancies if the first baby was well-grown, as long as the pregnancy is by the same father.
- Pregnancy complications should be explored. The symptom is far more significant if the pregnancy is complicated (see Clinical applications).

Physical examination

- Aimed at establishing the risk status of the pregnancy.
- Elevated blood pressure and proteinuria will signify pre-eclampsia complicating pregnancy.
- Symphysis–fundal height should be measured to assess fetal growth.
- Fetal movements may be palpable in the process of abdominal palpation.
- Excess amniotic fluid quantity can make maternal perception of fetal movements difficult.
- Demonstration of the fetal heart sounds is useful to reassure the parents. However, this is not clinically adequate to reassure fetal health.

Fetal assessment

Ultrasound examination for growth and liquor volume and, if needed, Doppler velocimetry should be arranged if no scan was done within the last 2 weeks.

- Ultrasound assessment is used to assess fetal growth and amniotic fluid volume.
- Doppler flow studies of the umbilical artery and the middle cerebral artery are useful indicators of uteroplacental insufficiency.
- At term and post-term a normal ultrasound assessment and fetal Doppler study do not exclude placental insufficiency. Fetal growth restriction is possible even if estimated fetal weight is within the normal range.
- Fetal biophysical profile is an assessment of current fetal status. Fetal hypoxia can be virtually excluded with a normal biophysical profile score.

Cardiotocography

Antenatal fetal heart rate monitoring is sometimes referred to as a 'non-stress test'.

- A reactive non-stress test is characterized by a normal baseline heart rate (110–160 bpm), normal baseline variability (5–25 bpm) at least 2 accelerations in a 20 min period, and absence of decelerations.
- The assessment of the fetal heart tracing is visual and subjective.
- A reactive non-stress test is a reliable sign of fetal well-being. However, it cannot predict future deterioration.
- Visual analysis of the fetal heart rate tracing is fraught with poor reproducibility.
- A computerized assessment eliminates subjective variation. It is objective, and the reproducibility is improved. Computerized CTG assessment is preferred over visual assessment using antenatal CTG.

Management

Management will depend on the underlying reason and perceived fetal risk. In a majority of cases, pregnancy assessment will be normal and reassurance is all that is needed. If the pregnancy is deemed to be at risk of fetal hypoxia, arrangements should be made for delivery. The route and timing of delivery will depend on the perceived severity of fetal compromise. Induction of labour may be advisable if it is easily possible, and fetal assessment is not grossly abnormal. Emergency Caesarean section may be required if the fetus is thought to be appreciably compromised.

Limitation of fetal movements as a sign of fetal well-being

Maternal perception of fetal movements indicates fetal well-being. However during the process of fetal response to placental insufficiency, fetal movements are one of the last parameters to become abnormal prior to intrauterine death. The time-window between cessation of fetal movements and stopping of heart activity is short. Presence of normal fetal movements has no prognostic capability. In acute situations such as placental abruption or cord prolapse, fetal movements may be a useless indicator of fetal well-being. In multiple pregnancy, fetal movements of the co-twin may be continued to be perceived, even after the other has suffered intrauterine demise.

☼ Abnormal antenatal fetal surveillance tests

The aim of antenatal fetal surveillance is to identify fetuses which are at risk of suffering intrauterine hypoxia with resultant damage, including death. This includes each and every pregnancy, as no pregnancy is free of this risk. However, experience from screening low-risk pregnant populations suggests that this approach does more harm than good when the risk of intrauterine hypoxia and the resultant sequel is low. Evidence suggests that fetal movement counting identifies fetuses at risk rather than improving outcome. Fundal height measurement has low prediction rate of identifying SGA fetuses at delivery. Primary step, therefore, is to identify those pregnancies, which are at a higher risk. Antenatal fetal surveillance is likely to be of benefit only in this group.

Biochemical tests

Maternal serum biochemistry, eg. oestriol and human placental lactogen are no longer used in clinical practice. A single unexplained elevated level of maternal serum alpha fetal protein in mid-trimester raises the risk of subsequent IUGR 5–10 fold.

Fetal movements

(See Chapter 4, pp. 96–97)

Ultrasound assessment

Fetal biometry
- Aimed at identifying fetal growth restriction.
- Fetal weight below the 10th centile is used as a criterion to identify small fetuses.
- Many fetuses with weight below 10th centile are normally grown but constitutionally small.
- Serial ultrasound measurements of the fetus is more accurate than clinical examination in the identification of small babies.
- Fetal abdominal circumference (AC) below the 5th centile is a sensitive indicator.
- Reduced amniotic fluid volume, and an advanced placental maturity are other contributory findings in growth restricted babies.

Placental dysfunction is indicated by reduced growth velocity, and increased resistance to flow in the umbilical artery.

Opposite is a typical ultrasound report of a fetus with growth restriction due to placental insufficiency.

Indication:
Growth restriction.

History:
Maternal age: 27 years, blood group: A positive.
Menstrual cycle irregular. Conception Ovulation drugs.

Gestational age:
27 weeks + 4 days (by ultrasound and LMP)

Growth scan:
Fetal measurements (plotted in relation to the normal mean ± 2 SDs).

Biparietal diameter (BPD)	66.0 mm	
Head circumference (HC)	219.9 m	
Abdominal circumference (AC)	164.9 mm	
Head/abdomen (HC/AC)	1.334	
Femur length (FL)	35.0 mm	
Est. fetal weight (Hadlock BPD -HC -AC -FL)	449 g	

Heart: action normal. Presentation: breech. Amniotic fluid: reduced.
Placenta: Anterior high, grannum Grade 3.

Fetal arterial and venous doppler flow study
Placental dysfunction is indicated by reduced growth velocity, and increased resistance to flow in the umbilical artery. There is redistribution of blood flow so that blood is selectively shunted to important organs like the brain and the heart, with less blood flow to less important organs like extremities, gastrointestinal tract, and skin. This is described as the 'head-sparing' effect or 'arterial redistribution'.

Normal umbilical artery waveforms
- The pregnancy is unlikely to develop loss of end-diastolic frequencies within a 7–10 day period, so that Doppler monitoring may be performed weekly.
- A growth-restricted fetus with normal umbilical artery waveforms will not be acidaemic, but has 10% chance of being hypoxaemic.
- Normal umbilical artery waveforms after 36 weeks gestation do not exclude fetal hypoxaemia and acidaemia.

Absent end-diastolic frequencies

- Loss of end-diastolic frequencies occurs only when over 75% of the placental vascular bed is obliterated. The latter is less likely to occur after 36 weeks gestation.
- Loss of end-diastolic frequencies is associated with an 85% chance that the fetus will be hypoxaemic and a 50% chance that it will also be acidaemic.
- Growth-restricted fetus with absent end-diastolic frequencies have a 4-fold increase in perinatal mortality compared to those with normal umbilical artery waveforms. The time between loss of end-diastolic frequencies and fetal death appears to differ for each fetus.
- Loss of end-diastolic frequencies precedes changes in the cardiotocograph by some days to weeks in growth-restricted fetuses.

Reversed end-diastolic frequencies

- Growth-restricted with reversed end-diastolic frequencies have a 10-fold increase in perinatal mortality compared to those with normal umbilical artery waveforms.
- Reversed frequencies in end-diastole are only observed in a few fetuses prior to death. This finding should be considered as a pre-terminal condition. Few, if any, fetuses will survive without delivery.

A typical report showing fetal blood flow redistribution is shown below.

Doppler:		
Umbilical artery:	PI 3.01	⊢——⊣ ▸
	End-diastolic flow: reverse flow	
Middle cerebral artery:	PI 1.63	⊢——⊣
	End-diastolic flow: positive	
Ductus venosus:	PIV 0.880	⊢——⊣
Diagnosis:		
SGA: likely uteroplacental insufficiency.		

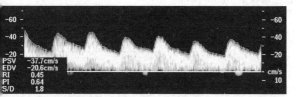

Fig. 4.1 Normal umbilical artery Doppler waveforms

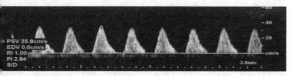

Fig. 4.2 Absent end-diastolic flow

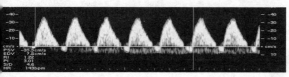

Fig. 4.3 Reversed end-diastolic flow

Biophysical profile (BPP)

The following criteria are assessed:

Fetal characteristic	Score 2	Score 0
Non-stress test	At least 2 episodes of fetal heart rate accelerations over 15 bpm lasting for more than 15 sec in 30 min.	Fewer than 2 episodes of fetal heart rate acceleration over 15 bpm lasting for more than 15 sec.
Fetal breathing movements	At least one episode of fetal breathing movements lasting more than 30 sec in a 30 min period.	Absent breathing movements or no episode of breathing lasting over 30 sec in 30 min.
Gross body movements	At least three fetal movements involving the fetal spine in a 30 min period.	2 or fewer movements in 30 min period.
Fetal tone	At least 1 episode of active fetal limb extension with a return to flexion in 30 min period. Opening and closing of the hand is considered as normal tone.	Slow extension with return to partial flexion, movements of limbs in full extension or absent limb movements.
Amniotic fluid volume	AFI between 5 cm and 25 cm.	AFI of below 5 cm or over 25 cm.

Several modifications of the score are used. A score of 8 or 10 is associated with excellent perinatal outcome. Scores of 4 and 6 are borderline, whereas scores of 0 or 2 are pathological. However there are some limitations:

- Requires access to expensive ultrasound equipment and trained operator.
- A normal BPP has limited prognostic value.
- Requires at least 30 min to complete.
- Lack of high quality evidence (randomized controlled trials) to show that BPP saves lives.
- The time interval between an abnormal BPP and fetal demise appears to be short.

Cardiotocography

Cardiotocography or electronic fetal heart rate monitoring was first applied during labor. Later its use was extended to the antenatal period in order to assess the fetal well-being even though it has no significant effect on perinatal outcome or interventions such as early elective delivery.

A recording of the fetal heart rate (FHR) pattern for a period of 20–30 min, called the nonstress test (NST), is one of the most widely used methods of antenatal fetal surveillance. A summary of the interpretation of the NST test is given below:

Antepartum cardiotocograph

Normal/reassuring/reactive

- At least 2 accelerations (>15 bpm for >15 sec) in 20 min, baseline heart rate 110–160 bpm, baseline variability 5–25 bpm, absence of decelerations.
- Sporadic decelerations amplitude <40 bpm are acceptable if duration <15 sec, <30 sec following an acceleration.
- When there is moderate tachycardia (160–180 bpm) or bradycardia (100–110 bpm), a reactive trace without decelerations is reassuring of good health.
- Interpretation/action—repeat according to clinical situation and the degree of fetal risk.

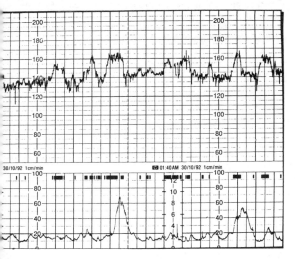

Fig. 4.4 Normal antenatal cardiotocograph

Suspicious/equivocal
- Absence of accelerations for >40 min (nonreactive).
- Baseline heart rate 160–180 bpm or 110–100 bpm.
- Reduced baseline variability (<5 bpm for >40 min).
- Baseline variability >25 bpm in the absence of accelerations.
- Sporadic decelerations of any type unless severe as described below.
- Interpretation/action—continue or repeat CTG within 24 hours, AFI, BPP, Doppler flow velocity waveform analysis.

Pathological/ominous
- Baseline heart rate <100 or >180 bpm.
- Reduced baseline variability <5 bpm for >90 min.
- Sinusoidal pattern (oscillation frequency <2–5 cycles/min, amplitude of >10 bpm for >40 min with no accelerations and no area of normal baseline variability).
- Repeated late, prolonged (>1 min) and severe variable (>40 bpm) decelerations.
- Interpretation/action—further evaluation (VAS, AFI, BPP, Doppler). Deliver if clinically appropriate.

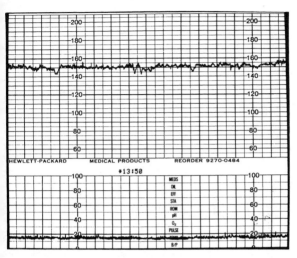

Fig. 4.5 Equivocal antenatal cardiotocograph—note reduced baseline variability and absence of accelerations

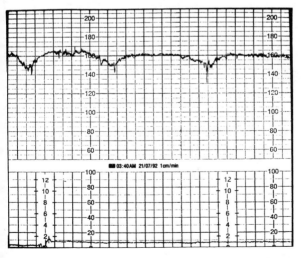

Fig. 4.6 Pathologial cardiotocograph with poor variability and decelerations

Intrapartum procedures and complications

Amarnath Bhide

Kevin Hayes and S. Arulkumaran

Leonie Penna

James Clarke

☠ Cord prolapse

Definition

Presence of cord below the presenting part is cord presentation when membranes are intact. Cord prolapse is when it prolapses through the cervix after membrane rupture. Occurs in approximately 1 : 600 deliveries with a cephalic presentation.

Predisposing factors

- Malpresentation
- Artificial rupture of membranes when the presenting part is un-engaged
- Prematurity including preterm pre-labour rupture of membranes
- Multiple pregnancy
- Polyhydramnios
- Intrauterine procedures such as placement of an intrauterine catheter for pressure monitoring or fluid infusion.

Diagnosis

Usually digital examination—cord pulsations can be felt by the examining fingers. Should be differentiated from maternal vessel pulsations, which can occasionally be felt. In case of fetal demise, pulsations may be absent. Only the cord can be felt.

Abnormal cardiotocography—deep variable decelerations, usually after history of membrane rupture. Cord prolapse should be suspected and ruled out.

Management

Immediate

- Call for help. Cord prolapse is an acute emergency, and quick response is of crucial importance.
- The examining hand should be retained in the same position to feel cord pulsations, and the presenting part should be elevated to prevent cord compression while the patient is being transferred to the theatre.
- It is important to keep the cord warm and moist by retaining it in the vagina. Exposure to the air outside leads to cord arterial spasm.
- Alternatively, filling the bladder with 500 ml saline may help to relieve cord compression at the pelvic brim.
- Additionally, Trendelenburg (head-down tilt) position can be given to relieve pressure on the head.
- Carry out a quick assessment of the gestational age, and ensure that it is a viable gestation.
- Administer facial oxygen.
- Uterine relaxants can be administered (terbutaline 250 micrograms by SC or IV route). The drug can cause hypotension and tachycardia, so contraindications (e.g. cardiac and hypertensive disease) should be ruled out.
- Alert theatre staff and anaesthetist.
- Neonatal crash call sent out.

Definitive
- Preparations should be made for immediate delivery. This involves an emergency Caesarean section under general anaesthetic in most cases.
- Possible exception is cord prolapse at full dilatation, or cord prolapse of the second twin after the delivery of the first baby. Instrumental delivery can be achieved, if safe and easily possible in singletons and twins with cephalic presentation. Breech extraction is possible in second of twins by an experienced obstetrician.
- Delivery of a hypoxic and depressed baby should be anticipated, and resuscitation facilities should be ready.
- Neonatologists should be present at delivery.

Debriefing
After the incident, the woman and the partner should receive adequate explanation of the sequence of events. They should be encouraged to ask any questions, as the steps taken from the time of diagnosis are too rapid to allow adequate explanations.

:☢: Abnormal fetal heart rate patterns in labour (prolonged decelerations)

Prolonged fetal deceleration of a fetal heart rate of < 80bpm for less than 3 min is considered as suspicious and <80 bpm for more than 3 min is considered as abnormal (NICE). Many cases will spontaneously resolve with no ill-effects.

Urgent delivery is required if it does not resolve as it significantly increases the risk of morbidity and mortality for the fetus.[†]

Associations

- Abnormal uterine activity (hyperstimulation)—commonly prostaglandin or oxytocin-induced but there may be no obvious cause
- Major placental abruption
- Uterine rupture
- Cord prolapse
- Following vaginal examination or artificial rupture of membranes
- Maternal hypotension (commonly post-epidural top up)
- Idiopathic.

Management

Points to consider

- Maternal/fetal risk factors (e.g. oxytocin use, previous LSCS, IUGR)
- CTG prior to bradycardia (normal/non-reassuring/pathological)—evidence has shown reduced variability pre-bradycardia has a higher chance of fetal acidaemia
- Presence or absence of regional anaesthesia
- Stage of labour (fully dilated or not).

Examine patient

- General observations (BP/pulse/temp)
- Interpret CTG **before** as well as now
- Abdominal and vaginal examination
- Maternal left lateral position (may improve uterine circulation)
- Exclude cord prolapse/abruption/uterine rupture—if one of the three proceed to immediate delivery
- Hyperstimulation—stop oxytocin and/or acute tocolysis
- Hypotension—fluid expansion and treat cause
- Alert appropriate staff (anaesthetist/ODA/paediatrician) if abruption, scar rupture or cord prolapse or prolonged deceleration >6 mins
- FBC/G&S (clotting ± crossmatching may be necessary)
- Maternal O_2 administration is of no proven benefit and is **not** recommended

---

[†] Ideally the unit should have a policy for category 1 or urgent (crash CS or code red) CS when there is immediate threat to the mother or baby. The aim is to deliver within 30 min. The midwife and doctor in the room should wheel the mother to OT and midwife in charge should activate the code to have OT staff, ODA, anaesthetist, and the paediatrician in the OT immediately in cases of abruption, cord prolapse, scar rupture, prolonged deceleration >6 min, scalp pH <7.20— the lower the pH, greater the urgency.

- In the presence of uterine hyperstimulation—stopping oxytocin and administration of a tocolytic agent (e.g. terbutaline 0.25 mg SC or slow IV when diluted in 5 ml saline) abolishes or reduces uterine contractions and allows the FHR to recover. This should be viewed as a temporary measure and should not delay delivery if the bradycardia does not resolve.

Aim is to deliver as soon as possible and an attempt should be made to fit the timescale below:
- 3 minutes—call obstetrician
- 6 minutes—prepare mother for delivery
- 9 minutes—go to theatre to prepare for LSCS or ventouse/forceps
- 12 minutes—deliver by quickest and safest method (usually LSCS)
- 15 minutes—complete delivery.

Maternal risks
- Operative delivery
- PPH[*]
- General anesthesia.

Fetal risks
- Asphyxia
- Death
- Meconium aspiration.

Resolution of bradycardia
- Spontaneous with subsequent normal CTG—continue monitoring
- Hyperstimulation with subsequent normal trace—continue monitoring, reduce or withhold oxytocin
- In presence of continuing CTG abnormalities—FBS (not within 10 min of bradycardia) or delivery as appropriate.

Outcome
- If delivered >20 min high risk of hypoxic ischaemic encephalopathy (HIE) and neonatal death (shorter time if prior CTG ominous ± meconium)
- Maternal and fetal outcome dependant upon underlying cause (e.g. major abruption/uterine rupture poorer outcome than cord prolapse)
- Maternal morbidity worse with GA.

---

[*] If a betamimetic is given and immediate delivery by CS is undertaken, PPH may ensue due to atonic uterus that does not respond to oxytocics. Propranolol 1 mg (a β-blocker) may be needed to reverse the betamimetic effect.

☠ Continuous abdominal pain in labour

Intermittent pain is a normal feature of labour. Continuous pain is never considered normal and is associated with several obstetric emergencies. The common use of epidural analgesia can make identification and diagnosis of the problem difficult and delayed.

Differential diagnosis
- Scar rupture
- Placental abruption
- Prolonged hypertonic contraction (hyperstimulation)
- Rare coincidental peritonism e.g. splenic rupture.

Scar rupture
Usually occurs in labour.

Associations
- Previous LSCS
- Previous myomectomy
- Previous cornual ectopic/hysterotomy/perforation
- Obstructed labour (especially multiparous)
- No apparent risk factors (especially in primips—subsequent history usually reveals previous uterine instrumentation e.g. unrevealed TOP).

Maternal risks
- Haemorrhage
- Hysterectomy
- Extension into adjacent tissues (bladder/ureters/broad ligament)
- Rarely death

Fetal risks
- Hypoxia
- Death

Symptoms and signs
- Change in pattern to continuous, severe pain
- Sessation of uterine contractions
- Brisk intrapartum PV bleeding
- Abnormal CTG (**prolonged and profound decelerations or sudden bradycardia which is the commonest FHR change or disappearance of FHR recording and difficulty in picking up the FHR**)
- Maternal tachycardia/hypotension
- Presenting part disappears out of pelvis
- Diffuse peritonism
- **Can be surprisingly subtle until there is significant blood loss—have a high index of suspicion if at risk e.g. trial of scar.**

Management

- Resuscitation with IV fluids/cross-match at least 4 units of blood stat.
- Immediate laparotomy, delivery of fetus and placenta within 15 min (by LSCS if still in the uterus) and repair of rupture site.
- Primary closure of rupture site with haemostasis is the main aim.
- Involvement of general, vascular, and urological surgeons may be necessary if extension occurs into ureters, bladder, broad ligament, or pelvic vessels.
- Immediate neonatal resuscitation will be necessary as the neonate is often in poor condition.
- Cord gases are mandatory.
- Fully document operative findings and event timings.
- Risk management form.

Subsequent pregnancies should always be delivered by elective LSCS at 37–38 weeks.

Placental abruption in labour

Associations
- History of APH
- PET ± IUGR
- Polyhydramnios (usually at time of ROM)
- All other risk factors for abruption.

Maternal risks
- Haemorrhage
- DIC
- Operative delivery
- Rhesus iso-immunization.

Fetal risks
- Hypoxia
- Death
- Exsanguination.

Symptoms and signs
- Usually sudden onset of severe, continuous pain.
- Sudden intrapartum PV bleeding is common (may be massive or unrevealed).
- Abnormal CTG (**prolonged bradycardia commonest**) or decelerations associated with too frequent contractions that indicate uterine irritability.
- Maternal tachycardia/hypotension.
- Rock hard, tender uterus.

Management
- Resuscitation with IV fluids/cross-match at least 4 units of blood stat.
- Blood for FBC and clotting (abruption can trigger DIC).
- Immediate LSCS delivery of fetus and placenta within 15 min if fetal bradycardia, abnormal FHR changes, uterine irritability, excessive bleeding, or haemodynamic disturbance (if fully dilated then Ventouse/forceps can be considered).

- Replace blood loss with whole blood (group-specific if necessary).
- Haematological advice about replacement of clotting factors and/or platelets if required.
- Needs HDU care with strict fluid balance and senior obstetric and anaesthetic input (especially if have underlying PET).
- Immediate neonatal resuscitation will be necessary as the neonate is often in poor condition.
- Cord gases are mandatory.
- Fully document operative findings and event timings.
- Risk management form.

☢: Instrumental delivery for fetal distress in the second stage of labour

'Fetal distress' is the second commonest cited indication for instrumental delivery in the second stage of labour after prolonged second stage. 'Fetal distress' is often poorly defined. Fetal pH falls quicker in the second stage so delivery should be completed within 20–30 min of decision to deliver for 'fetal distress'.

If, in the presence of fetal distress, a difficult vaginal delivery is anticipated then serious consideration should be given to emergency LSCS instead.

Indications for instrumental delivery for fetal distress

• Prolonged bradycardia
• Pathological CTG
• Non-reassuring CTG with fresh meconium or abnormal FBS results
• Acute event e.g. abruption, cord prolapse.

Prerequisites for safe instrumental delivery

• Informed consent
• Full dilatation
• No more than 0–1/5ths palpable abdominally
• Presenting part at the level of the ischial spines or lower
• Position defined (e.g. OA, OT, OP)
• Empty bladder
• Adequate analgesia (epidural, pudendal and/or local infiltration)
• Examination *must* be carried out by the most senior obstetrician available.

Never accept somebody else's examination findings when you are performing the delivery.

Choice of Instrument

Choose the instrument that will best achieve a timely delivery.
• Different practitioners have a preference for ventouse or forceps.
• Forceps (non-rotational)—less chance of failure, more maternal pain and trauma.
• Ventouse—less pain and maternal trauma, more chance of failure.
• Forceps (rotational)—only defensible in experienced hands, LSCS usually preferable.

Action

• Decision to deliver (aim for 20 min for completion, 15 for prolonged bradycardia)
• **Call for help** (anaesthetist/ODA/paediatrician/lead midwife)
• Obtain consent (preferably written but verbal will suffice)
• In the event of an acute event e.g. abruption—FBC + clotting/cross-match/IV access
• Ensure all prerequisites are met
• Move to theatre promptly for trial of instrumental delivery (in delivery room only if 'easy lift out')

- Reassess whole situation ('Should I be doing a LSCS?')
- Choose instrument and attempt delivery ('3 pulls and you are out'—no descent with 3 judicious pulls, abandon procedure)
- **If you fail to deliver with your first choice instrument then quick resort to LSCS is usually advisable, unless the head is seen at the perineum and needs a lift out. Evidence has shown that use of ventouse *and* forceps has a poorer neonatal outcome.**
- Continuous fetal monitoring throughout the procedure is useful.
- Timekeeping is essential
- If successful delivery, baby is handed straight to paediatricians
- Cord gases are mandatory
- Risk management form should be completed in the case of adverse outcome to the fetus or mother
- Full, contemporaneous documentation
- Counsel parents and explain sequence of events regardless of outcome.

☠ Shoulder dystocia

Difficulty with delivery of the fetal shoulders, after delivery of the head with the need for *another procedure* to effect delivery.

Shoulder dystocia is rare, largely unpredictable, and associated with increased maternal morbidity and increased perinatal morbidity and mortality. It is a true emergency where every second counts and remaining calm and judicious of action is vital. Litigation is common when neonatal outcome is poor or there is evidence of injury.

Reported incidences vary from 1:50–1:500 deliveries (poorly defined and highly subjective).

Associations
- Previous shoulder dystocia
- Macrosomia (particularly >4.5 kg),
- Maternal obesity
- Diabetic pregnancy
- Slow progress (7–10 cm)
- Use of syntocinon,
- Operative e.g. forceps/ventouse delivery

The majority of cases however occur with no risk factors and are in babies <4.5 kg. Prediction is therefore difficult but the single best predictor is previous shoulder dystocia.

Maternal risk
- Genital tract trauma
- 3rd and 4th degree tears
- PPH
- Poor birth experience

Fetal risk
- Death
- Asphyxia
- Brachial plexus injury
  (Erb's/Klumpke palsy 5–15%)
- Fractured clavicle/humerus (10–15%)

Management
Understanding the problem—this is a *bony* dystocia commonly anterior shoulder on symphysis ± posterior shoulder on sacral promontory. All subsequent manoeuvres aim to *increase the pelvic space* available or *rotate* the shoulder to dislodge it. Overzealous traction on the fetal head causes injury and should be avoided.

Algorithm for the management of shoulder dystocia: HELPERR[1]
- **H**elp—most senior midwife and obstetrician/anaesthetist/ paediatrician/health care assistants.
- **E**valuate for episiotomy—increases room available for further manoeuvres.

[1] HELPERR algorithm first described on the ALSO course. (www.also.org.uk).

- **L**egs (McRoberts manoeuvre)—hyperflexion of thighs onto abdomen increases the 'pelvic space' available.
- **P**ressure (directed suprapubic)—aims to rotate anterior shoulder forward off symphysis.
- **E**nter the pelvis (Wood's screw manoeuvre)—aims to internally rotate anterior shoulder to become posterior and bring the new 'anterior' shoulder below symphysis in a 'corkscrew' fashion.
- **R**emove posterior arm—posterior arm flexed and swept over fetal chest to exteriorize and then perform rotation as above.
- **R**oll onto all fours—change in position may improve pelvic diameters and space available.

The majority of babies will be delivered by the end of the algorithm.

If these fail then it is recommended that they are *repeated* before moving on to further procedures including:

- Cephalic replacement (Zavanelli procedure) and LSCS—has been successfully described.
- Symphysiotomy—not recommended unless knowledge and skill available due to maternal morbidity.
- Cleidotomy—deliberate fracture of the fetal clavicles usually only if the fetus is dead.

Preventing asphyxia and death
Fetal pH may fall by 0.04 per min. Delivery within 5 min (pH fall of 0.2) is usually associated with a good outcome if the fetus has a normal pH to begin with.

After delivery
- Anticipate PPH and act accordingly
- Evaluate thoroughly for 3rd/4th degree tears
- Cord blood gases must be taken
- Fully document all actions including accurate timings
- Fill out risk management form
- Counsel parents
- Arrange follow-up at 6 weeks to discuss events and subsequent pregnancies.

Prevention and counselling
Shoulder dystocia is largely unpredictable. The vast majority of women with previous shoulder dystocia will not subsequently suffer it (reported repeat incidence of 1–16%).

Elective CS for women with previous shoulder dystocia *and* diabetes *and/or* whose babies suffered an injury last time is recommended as recurrence is higher. Full explanation of the pros and cons of elective CS or trial of vaginal delivery will help a woman decide mode of delivery in a subsequent pregnancy. Induction of labour at around 37–38 weeks for women with risk factors has **not** been shown to reduce the incidence of shoulder dystocia and is not recommended.

☼ Acute tocolysis

Indications
- Acute fetal distress (prolonged bradycardia) especially with uterine hyperstimulation
- Cord prolapse
- Fetal entrapment during delivery especially for a second twin (e.g. need for internal or external version)
- Transverse lie at time of CS—esp. preterm, dorso-inferior with ruptured membranes
- Preterm breech at CS especially for the after coming head
- Retained placenta that has separated
- Replacement of uterine inversion.

Aims of acute tocolysis
- Induce uterine relaxation to allow adequate fetal perfusion and return of normal fetal heart rate.
- Possibly achieve a better fetal pH at delivery (intrauterine resuscitation).
- Increase the time available for urgent delivery without fetal asphyxia (e.g. preparation for delivery, opening a second theatre, use of regional anaesthesia vs GA).
- Allow easier access and fetal manipulation in a difficult delivery.
- Allow easier uterine manipulation.

Acute tocolysis drugs
Many agents have been used including salbutamol, terbutaline, ritodrine, ethanol, glycerol trinitrate (GTN), nifedipine, magnesium sulphate, hexoprenaline and atosiban.

Management
- Treat underlying causes e.g. stop or reduce oxytocin if hyperstimulation present.
- Prepare for urgent delivery if fetal bradycardia or cord prolapse (usually LSCS).
- Make appropriate plans depending upon the indications above.
- Terbutaline 0.25 mg in 5 ml saline IV over 5 min (or 0.25 mg SC) has been shown to reduce uterine activity and improve both fetal heart rates and subsequent cord pH, including continuing labour and achieving vaginal delivery. Maternal side effects include palpitations, tachycardia, and hypotension. The maximal effect lasts for 20–30 min. If CS was performed, there is threat of atonic PPH. Propanalol 1 mg IV needs to be given to reverse the effect and for oxytocin to be effective.
- Salbutamol 8 puffs inhaled via a spacing device is not effective in relaxing the uterus. Ritodrine 6 mg in 10 ml saline IV over 2–3 mins has also been used.
- β-adrenergics are particularly useful in cases of hyperstimulation but may even be beneficial without hyperstimulation.

- GTN 5 mg in 100 ml saline (50 µg/ml) IV—initial dose 200 µg repeated at 1–2 min intervals as required has also been used extensively. IV use has a more predictable uterine response than the sublingual aerosol spray (400 µg) and is preferred if available. The uterine response is rapid and short lasting (1–2 min) and may therefore need repeating. Maternal side effects include flushing and hypotension. The effect is rapidly reversible with oxytocin.
- Atosiban has been used extensively for non-acute tocolysis but could be used in acute situations.

Acute tocolytic use for fetal distress should be considered as a temporary measure and unless the fetal heart rate returns to normal delivery should be expedited urgently.

Contraindications to tocolysis

- Maternal hypotension
- Maternal haemorrhage or hypovolaemia
- Moderate/severe maternal cardiac disease.

☠ Symphysiotomy and destructive operations

Symphysiotomy

Symphisiotomy is the surgical division of the fibrocartilaginous symphysis pubis to open the pelvis. It is very rarely performed nowadays but still has a place in the management of certain obstetric emergencies particularly in the developing world.

Indications
- Mild—moderate obstructed labour where Caesarean delivery may be inappropriate.
- Severe shoulder dystocia unresponsive to all other attempts at delivery.
- Trapped after-coming head in a vaginal breech delivery.

Contraindications
- Severe cephalo-pelvic disproportion
- Transverse lie
- Major pelvic deformity.

Procedure
1. Only to be undertaken by an experienced practitioner.
2. Adequate anaesthesia (GA, regional, or local infiltration with opiate sedation).
3. Place in lithotomy position with 2 assistants holding the legs.
4. Catheterization of the bladder to identify the urethra, and empty the bladder, and retain rigid plastic or metal catheter in situ.
5. Identify the symphysis and make a stab incision through the skin and the symphysis cartilage just below the upper border and rotate the scalpel upwards to cut the lower fibres using the upper fibres as a fulcrum.
6. Remove the scalpel and insert it at the same point but with the blade facing upwards to extend the incision up to fully divide the symphysis (this causes less morbidity than partial division and forced abduction). With two fingers in the vagina help to push the urethra sideways and to allow judgement on how far to incise.
7. Deal with original indication for symphysiotomy.
8. Episiotomy is recommended as the anterior vaginal wall is unsupported and tension on it can lead to avulsion and urethral damage.
9. Antibiotic prophylaxis recommended.
10. Evaluate for urethral or bladder injury.
11. Suture incision edges to achieve haemostasis.
12. Orthopaedic and physio input is vital.
13. Bladder drainage for 48 hours is recommended.
14. Physical support of the pelvis is the mainstay of treatment to aid healing.
15. Discharge is appropriate once ambulation is confident.

Risks
- Pain
- Haemorrhage

- Urethral and/or bladder injury
- Osteitis pubis and retropubic abscess
- Long term pain and pelvic instability. May need plating with orthopaedic help.

The procedure is increasingly hard to justify in the developed world. It should be seen as a last resort and only carried out by people experienced in the procedure or in settings where abdominal delivery carries higher risks.

Destructive operations

These are performed to remove the fetus and placenta piecemeal in the presence of fetal death or futile outcome where spontaneous vaginal delivery may not be possible and/or abdominal delivery is to be avoided. These procedures are increasingly rarely performed and should only be carried out by an experienced practitioner. In the developed world CS is almost always preferred.

Indications

- Severe obstructed labour with fetal death (by far the commonest indication)
- Severe or lethal fetal abnormality obstructing vaginal delivery
- After severe shoulder dystocia in the event of fetal death
- After head entrapment in a breech vaginal delivery with fetal death.

Procedure

1. General anaesthesia is generally recommended.
2. Aseptic technique required.
3. Sufficient dilatation of the cervix is required, usually fully dilated, but is possible >7 cm.
4. Percutaneous drainage of any large cystic structures e.g. cystic hygroma may facilitate delivery.
5. Craniotomy involves a cruciate incision through a suture line with either a blunt forceps or sharp scissors followed by extraction of the brain tissue. The head can than be delivered by attaching Kocher forceps to the cranium and pulling down.
6. Decapitation may be used for transverse lies to facilitate vaginal removal.
7. Evisceration may also be required for the abdomen and chest where decompression is necessary to achieve delivery.
8. Cleidotomy to reduce the bi-acromial diameter may be required if there are impacted shoulders.
9. Haemorrhage should be anticipated and prevented with liberal use of oxytocics.
10. Antibiotic cover is also recommended to reduce sepsis in the puerperium.
11. Full counselling should be available for patients and staff as these procedures can be highly traumatic.

Risks

- Haemorrhage
- Infection
- Uterine perforation
- Psychological morbidity for patients and staff.

:O: Twin delivery

It is very important to try to establish chorionicity in all twins during the antenatal period, as this will influence labour management. Ideally this requires an ultrasound scan prior to 16 weeks gestation, as after this gestation ultrasound is known to be less accurate.

Common points of management

- Survival rates for preterm twins are lower than for equivalent gestation singletons. Urgent review by an experienced neonatologist is essential to assist with management in all cases of twins at high risk of preterm delivery especially in deciding whether very early gestation (24–26 weeks) should be managed expectantly rather than undergoing operative delivery such as CS.
- Steroids should be administered (2 doses of betamethasone 12mg IM 24 hours apart) where there is a significant chance of preterm delivery.
- Tocolytic agents can be used in cases of spontaneous preterm labour (cervix <4 cm) to allow maximum benefit from steroid administration. Atosiban or nifedipine should be used.
- Hypertensive disorders (including pre-eclampsia), acute fatty liver, obstetric cholestasis, abruption, and placenta praevia more commonly complicate twin pregnancies and should always be considered even in non-specific presentations.
- Previous CS is not an absolute indication for repeat CS in an uncomplicated twin pregnancy.

Monochorionic monoamniotic (MCMA) twins

- Advise delivery by CS due to the risk of cord entanglement and malpresentation of second twin during delivery.
- Elective delivery at 32–34 weeks (after prophylactic steroids) is recommended due to the risk of sudden intra-uterine death of one or both twins from a cord accident due to entanglement.
- At viable gestations emergency CS should be performed in established preterm labour.

Monochorionic diamniotic (MCDA) twins

Mode and timing of delivery remains controversial due to a paucity of data relating delivery mode and gestation to outcome. However, some obstetricians recommend caesarean delivery to avoid the risk of acute twin–twin transfusion syndrome (TTTS) during labour or after delivery of first twin (thus compromising second twin).

Delivery at 36 weeks is sometimes recommended to avoid the risk of worsening TTTS in the late 3rd trimester. Pregnacies which have no evidence of TTTS, or where a laser has successfully treated TTTS can be managed as per dichorionic diamniotic (DCDA) twins.

The following should be considered as indication for planned caesarean delivery:

- Any evidence of TTTS during pregnancy (growth discrepancy >10%, discrepancy in amniotic fluid volume (AFV), abnormal fetal Dopplers) not successfully treated by laser ablation of communicating vessels.

- Non-cephalic leading twin.
- Maternal request for CS.
- Any of the above in early labour (including preterm labour at a viable gestation).

Dichorionic diamniotic (DCDA) twins

Antenatal care plan should have been made in consultation with the parents resulting in a plan for delivery. The following should be considered as indication for planned caesarean delivery:

- Non-cephalic leading twin
- Severe growth restriction in either twin
- Either of the above in preterm labour at a viable gestation
- Maternal request
- Any of the above in early labour at term.

On admission in labour:

- Check gestation (review ultrasound scans)
- Review ultrasound for evidence of fetal growth and well-being
- Fetal hearts simultaneously (twin cardiotocograph)
- Presentation of twin 1 (ultrasound if necessary)
- Cervical dilation
- Plans made for delivery prior to labour
- Presentation of twin 2 can be checked but is not relevant to decision regarding mode of delivery as even a cephalic twin 2 may move to a breech presentation (and vice versa).

Vaginal twin delivery

Recommendations for all women planning vaginal birth and for women with uncomplicated twins who were requesting LSCS now in advanced labour (>6 cm).

Management:

- Discuss analgesia. Epidural is not mandatory but should be recommended to avoid the discomfort associated with any manipulation that may be required to assist in delivering twin 2 and to avoid the maternal risk of general anaesthetic should emergency CS be required.
- Discuss fetal monitoring and recommend continuous electronic fetal monitoring for both twins simultaneously to allow early detection of fetal heart rate abnormality.
- Recommend intravenous cannulation and send blood for haemoglobin and G&S.
- Give ranitidine 150 mg PO 8 hourly during labour due to increase risk of Caesarean delivery.
- *First stage* of labour managed as per a singleton fetus:
  - Oxytocin augmentation may be used (standard dose protocols for singleton).
- *Second stage:*
  - Twin 1 delivered as per singleton (spontaneous, ventouse or forceps).
  - Immediately post-delivery of twin 1, check lie of twin 2 by palpation (ultrasound if required) and ensure the fetal heart is monitored effectively.

- If lie is non-longitudinal attempt external version to cephalic (or breech) prior to the onset of contractions.
- Await onset of contractions. If not already running, an intravenous oxytocin infusion can be considered if there are no contractions after 10 min.
- Encourage active pushing with contractions when presenting part enters pelvis.
- Do not rupture membranes until presenting part is within pelvis and contractions have re-established.
- If fetal heart rate becomes abnormal, expedite delivery as required (CS, high ventouse, breech extraction depending on clinical circumstances and experience of operator).
- If fetal heart remains normal await decent of presenting part into the pelvis for up to 1 hour. Beyond this time intervention to expedite delivery is required (CS, high ventouse, breech extraction depending on clinical circumstances and experience of operator).
- Ventouse may be performed with a cervix that is fully dilated or with dilatation of 8–9 cm and with the head above the ischial spines for delivery of twin 2 *only*. Care must be taken to ensure maternal tissues are not caught during cup application and that the cup is applied as close as possible to the flexion point on the fetal scalp.
- See comments in Breech delivery (p.130) regarding breech extraction.
- *Third stage:*
  - Recommend active management with bolus of oxytocic given with delivery of twin 2 (IM syntometrine or IM/IV syntocinon 5 units) followed by an oxytocin (syntocinon) infusion 5–10 units/hour for 4–6 hours

Caesarean delivery for twins

- Twin 1 is usually delivered without difficulty as per a singleton.
- Avoid rupturing the membranes of twin 2 until the head or breech is palpated in the uterine incision. Delivery can be expedited by feeling for a fetal foot through the intact membranes and gently pulling it into the uterine incision. This is often required if twin 2 is lying transverse. An intravenous oxytocin infusion (syntocinon 10 units/hour) should be used following delivery of twin 2 to reduce the risk of post-partum haemorrhage.

Preterm twin delivery (<34 weeks)

Diagnosis

- Confirm gestation, chorionicity, last presentation, and fetal growth patterns from previous ultrasound scans if available.
- Check presentation of twin 1 (ultrasound if necessary).
- Try to establish diagnosis of labour (but avoid digital vaginal examination if ruptured membranes unless mother appears to be in established labour).
- Consider sterile speculum examination to assess in possible early labour.

Investigations
- Vaginal swab
- Check white cell count and C-reactive protein
- Estimate fetal weights if appropriate expertise available
- Simultaneous cardiotocograph on a twin monitor.

Management
- See general comments and delivery mode comments specific to chorionicity.
- Vaginal delivery may be considered in early gestations (24–26 weeks) in circumstances where Caesarean would be recommended at a more advanced gestation (e.g. breech twin 1) as survival chances are lower regardless of mode of delivery.
- Remember antibiotic prophylaxis for group B streptococcus (GBS).

Intra-uterine death (IUD) of one twin

Check chorionicity from previous ultrasound scans prior to discussion of risk to the surviving fetus with the parents.

Dichorionic twins
- Risk to the surviving twin is related to the risk of preterm labour (and thus gestation at diagnosis of IUD).
- Manage conservatively unless abruption is the likely cause of death.

All monochorionic (MCDA, MCMA) twins
- 25% risk of death or neurological handicap due to hypotensive episodes at the time of death of the co-twin plus the risk of preterm labour.
- If recent death and gestation >34 weeks recommend delivery to reduce risk long-term mortality or morbidity to surviving twin.
- If death occurred >24 hours ago manage conservatively unless abruption is the likely cause of death.
- <34 weeks gestation administer steroids (betamethasone ×2 doses 24 hours apart) and continue conservative management:
  - continuous CTG if immediately post-death of twin.
  - arrange serial ultrasound to monitor fetal brain development in surviving twin.
- If conservative management deliver as per singleton (gestation and delivery mode).
- If cause of death was abruption and there is evidence of uterine irritability, bleeding, or abnormal FHR, delivery may need to expedited by the appropriate route.

Triplet delivery
- Expertise in vaginal delivery of triplets is uncommon. Most units deliver triplets at viable gestations by CS.
- Triplet pregnancy is often complicated by severe pre-eclampsia.
- Elective delivery at 34 weeks is often recommended to reduce the need for emergency intra-partum Caesarean delivery.
- 20% of women with triplets will labour prior to 32 weeks gestation.
- Steroids and tocolysis should be administered as for singletons.
- Discussion with an experienced neonatologist is essential in all cases of preterm labour.

:Ö: **Breech delivery**

Since the publication of the Canadian term breech study, many obstetricians recommend delivery of the term breech diagnosed prior to labour by elective CS. There remain a number of situations where vaginal breech delivery will be required and it is therefore essential that departments are prepared for this situation. As vaginal breech delivery is now less common, skills must be gained and maintained by the use of mannequins and with aids such as videos.

Planning delivery mode

Vaginal breech delivery should be considered in:
- Any woman with a breech presentation first diagnosed in active labour
- Woman counselled regarding the risks of vaginal breech delivery antenatally who wish to pursue the option of vaginal breech delivery
- Women planned for elective Caesarean admitted prior to surgery in advanced labour (>6 cm)
- Preterm labour with breech presentation
- Second twin.

Recommend caesarean delivery in the following:
- Footling breech
- Extended fetal neck on antenatal ultrasound
- History of previous difficult vaginal delivery
- Estimated fetal weight above 4000 g
- Fetal heart rate abnormality in early labour.

Diagnosis
- Abdominal palpation
- Vaginal examination:
  - station
  - fetal sacral position
  - attitude of breech:
    1. footling (buttocks not within pelvis only feet)
    2. flexed (buttocks in pelvis with feet palpable along side)
    3. extended (buttocks only in pelvis, feet not palpable)

Urgent issues
- Risk of cord prolapse if footling breech and ruptured membranes.
- Cord compression is more common in breech presentation which may result in the fetus becoming hypoxic during labour.

Investigations
- Ultrasound scan on labour ward to confirm diagnosis if breech presentation is suspected in early labour and vaginal examination is inconclusive
- Cardiotocograph for contractions and fetal well-being
- Take blood for haemoglobin and G&S (risk of emergency caesarean)

Management during 1st stage
- Advise fluid-only during labour.
- Recommend and establish IV access.
- Give anti-emetic (e.g. metoclopramide 10 mg PO or slow IV) and antacid (e.g. ranitidine 150mg PO).
- Inform anaesthetist.
- Epidural is recommended for pain relief (in case 2nd stage intervention required) but is not mandatory. A pudendal block can be used as an alternative. Spinal anaesthesia is best avoided as it prevents effective pushing which is essential for safe breech delivery.
- Assess progress 2–4 hourly throughout labour and expect progress 0.5–1 cm/hour.
- Amniotomy is only required if progress is sub-optimal. If progress is normal, membranes should be left intact, as this will reduce the incidence of cord compression decelerations.
- Oxytocin augmentation may be considered in primigravid women for poor progress. In multigravid women oxytocin is not recommended unless contraction frequency is sub-optimal (<4 in 10 min)
- Fetal heart rate abnormality should be managed by standard protocols. Fetal blood sampling from the buttocks can be considered. Meconium should not be assumed to be due to the breech presentation and requires careful review prior to the 2nd stage.
- Theatre facilities should be available nearby in case CS is required. This avoids the need to transfer to theatre for the 2nd stage if labour is progressing normally.

Management during 2nd stage
- An individual experienced in vaginal breech delivery should supervise delivery.
- Most obstetricians prefer breech delivery with the woman in a dorsal/recumbent position, however, breech delivery on all fours appears to be safe. Standing breech delivery should be avoided.
- Regardless of delivery position facilities for lithotomy should be available (poles or manual assistance).
- Commence active pushing when the buttocks are visible or one hour after diagnosis of full dilatation (whichever is sooner). However pushing should not be commenced until the breech has reached the level of the ischial spines.
- Accoucher should adopt a 'hands-off' approach to delivery of the breech. The breech may be supported as it descends but traction should *never* be used, as this will increase the risk of nuchal arms and extension of the neck.
- Breech extraction describes the procedure where the membranes are ruptured when the breech is high in the pelvis or above the pelvic brim, a limb is pulled down into the vagina with traction continued to facilitate delivery. As this is associated with a high neonatal morbidity and mortality, it should only be considered if caesarean delivery cannot (or should not) be undertaken for some reason. Likewise it may be tempting to apply traction to the groins of an extended breech or to the limbs of a flexed breech if there is poor progress or a serious

fetal heart abnormality but delivery by Caesarean should be undertaken even at this late stage to avoid fetal risk.

- When the body has delivered to the level of the lower border of the scapula there is likely to be severe cord compression resulting in a rapidly developing fetal hypoxia. Delivery of the shoulders and head will normally occur rapidly and spontaneously but assistance may be required if there is delay of more than 2–3 min.

- It is important to ensure adequate contractions to achieve rapid delivery. If contractions become less frequent in the 2nd stage an oxtocin infusion should be commenced or the option of CS considered.

- Low apgar scores are more common following breech delivery and an individual experienced in neonatal resuscitation should be available at the time of delivery.

- Interventions that may be employed but will not be necessary in all cases:
  - *Support to* maintain fetus in sacro-anterior position (hold the baby at the hips as pressure on the abdomen can cause damage).
  - *Gentle flexion* of the knees (pressure in popliteal fossa) in an extended breech to allow the legs to deliver.
  - *Episiotomy* (only after anus has delivered over posterior fourchette to reduce risk of perineal tears and to facilitate delivery).
  - *Lovset's manoeuvre* to deliver the arms if these are extended (they should deliver without manipulation otherwise).
    — turn baby in a half a circle, keeping the back uppermost, applying downward traction at the same time, so that the posterior arm becomes anterior and delivers under the pubic arch. To deliver the other arm repeat the procedure turning the baby back in a half circle.
  - *Assist head delivery* in a slow and controlled way once the nape of the neck is clearly visible:
    1. *Mauriceau-Smellie Veit manoeuvre* is especially useful in multigravida
       — Place baby with body over accoucher's arm, place the first and third fingers of hand on cheekbones and second finger in the mouth to pull the jaw down and flex the head.
       or
    2. *Forceps* to the after-coming head. An assistant is required to hold baby whilst the forceps are applied (care must be taken not to over extend the neck).
  - *Insertion* of a weighted speculum into the vagina (if there is delay in delivery of the head may allow breathing).

Indications for secondary caesarean section

- Pathological fetal heart rate pattern at any stage in labour unless fetal blood sampling is normal (caesarean delivery is appropriate up to the point where the scapula becomes visible—see comments about breech extraction above).
- Failure of progress in 1st stage of labour.

- Inadequate contractions in the 2nd stage where oxytocin is considered inappropriate.
- Failure of the breech to descend to the level of the ischial spines (passive 2nd stage).
- Failure of the breech to descend to delivery of the buttocks after one hour active 2nd stage.

⑦ **Abnormal lie/presentation in labour**

Transverse lie in labour
Causes
- Obstruction in pelvis
  - fibroid in the lower segment
  - large ovarian cyst
  - placenta praevia.
- Fetal abnormality
  - hydrocephalus,
  - neuromuscular problems (and chromosome abnormality).
- Increased uterine capacity
  - multiparity (especially grand multiparity due to lax uterus)
  - preterm gestation
  - polyhydramnios especially with non-macrosomic baby.

Diagnosis
- On palpation—no presenting part in pelvis, fetal poles palpable laterally.
- On vaginal examination presenting part is not reached, fetal limbs or back palpable.
- Fibroid or cystic mass may be palpable (abdominal or vaginal examination).
- Concurrent ante-partum haemorrhage suggests placenta praevia (vaginal examination contraindicated)
- Confirm labour—uterine contraction present and vaginal examination reveals cervical effacement and dilatation >3 cm.

Urgent issues
- Rupture of membranes may result in cord prolapse (less likely if fetus is with the back down).
- If contractions are strong (advanced labour) in a multigravid woman there is a risk of uterine rupture as the labour may get obstructed. This is especially true if there is a uterine scar and immediate delivery must be undertaken.

Investigations
- Review previous ultrasound scan reports for possible cause.
- Ultrasound scan on labour ward to confirm diagnosis and look for causes.
- Cardiotocograph for contractions and fetal wellbeing.
- Take blood for G&S, FBC.

Management
- Keep nil by mouth.
- Recommend and establish intravenous access.
- Give anti-emetic (metoclopramide 10 mg PO or slow IV) and antacid (ranitidine 150 mg PO).
- Inform anaesthetist and theatre team.
- If evidence of obstruction in pelvis delivery by immediate CS is required.

- If no evidence of obstruction and membranes are intact, attempt external version to a cephalic presentation between contractions. If successful, controlled amniotomy can be considered whilst lie is maintained by a second operator. Due to the risk of cord prolapse this should be performed with facilities for immediate CS available.
- If no evidence of obstruction but membranes have ruptured, internal podalic version to breech could be considered at the limits of fetal viability (23–25 weeks gestation) but at other gestations immediate delivery by CS is likely to be safer for the fetus.

Prior to caesarean section remember:

- Consent for removal if ovarian cyst.
- For suspected placenta praevia cross-match blood and request senior obstetrician to be present.
- Caesarean delivery of transverse fetus with back down can be difficult especially after membrane rupture, therefore aim to perform internal version to breech during Caesarean before rupturing membranes. If membranes have ruptured consider performing vertical uterine incision (De Lee) particularly for preterm gestations.
- Consider use of bolus dose of tocolytics to facilitate atraumatic delivery.

Brow presentation

A brow presentation occurs when there is poor flexion of the fetal head. This results in a much bigger presenting diameter and an average baby at term will not deliver vaginally. Smaller and preterm infants may deliver without flexion as a brow but in larger babies vaginal delivery will only be possible if the head flexes to an occipito-anterior or occipito posterior position or extends to become a face presentation (see pp.136–7). Good contractions are required to facilitate this flexion. However if flexion fails to occur, the labour becomes obstructed and there is a risk of uterine rupture if the contractions are strong.

Causes

- Fetal abnormality (any resulting in an inability for good neck flexion)
- Poor uterine activity
- Preterm gestations
- In most cases no cause can be identified.

Diagnosis

- Diagnosis in early labour is unusual
- Abdominal palpation shows a non-engaged head
- Palpation of orbital ridges during vaginal examination.

Urgent issue

In women with a uterine scar (previous CS) immediate delivery by CS should be considered if the diagnosis of brow presentation is made in established labour at term due to the risk of scar dehiscence if the labour is obstructed.

Management
- Assess gestation and estimate fetal weight as low birth weight infant is likely to deliver spontaneously even if abnormal presentation persists.
- Assess contractions:
  - good contractions are required to facilitate flexion of the fetal neck.
  - commence oxytocin infusion in primigravid women with slow progress regardless of contraction pattern but only in multigravid women with slow progress and inadequate contraction pattern (less than 4 in 10 min).
- Assess and monitor progress in labour.
  - brow presentation in early labour is more likely to resolve than when diagnosis is made in advanced labour.
  - remember risk of uterine rupture if contractions are strong and the head does not flex (especially in multigravid women).
  - delivery should be by CS following failure of normal cervical dilatation in the 1st stage of labour or failure of flexion and decent of the head on active pushing in the 2nd stage of labour.
  - assisted vaginal delivery by forceps or Ventouse is not possible, if spontaneous flexion does not occur delivery by Caesarean will be required.
- Give ranitidine 150 mg PO and limit oral intake due to risk of Caesarean delivery.
- Recommend epidural for pain-relief after diagnosis (increased risk of CS).
- Monitor fetal heart rate
  - fetal blood sampling is not recommended for fetal heart rate abnormality (deliver by CS).

Face presentation

A face presentation occurs when instead of flexion the fetal head becomes fully extended. The diameter of the average fetal head is such that this presentation can deliver vaginally. However the face is a poor cervical dilatator and thus good contractions are required, and even then progress will often be slow. As the head delivers across the perineum by flexion in this presentation, a fetus that moves into a mento posterior position cannot deliver vaginally as flexion will be prevented by the symphysis-pubis.

Causes
- Fetal abnormality resulting in poor fetal tone or neck hyper-extension such as thyroid tumour or anencephaly
- Relative cephalopelvic disproportion (large baby or small pelvis)
- Grand multiparity
- In most cases no cause can be identified.

Diagnosis
- Abdominal palpation is usually unremarkable if the head is engaged
- Smooth rounded occiput may be palpable on the opposite side of the fetal body if the head is not engaged
- On vaginal examination the fetal eyes, nose bridge, and mouth can be palpated. Oedema in soft tissues may lead to the mistaken diagnosis of a breech presentation
- Diagnosis in early labour is difficult.

Management

- Review antenatal ultrasound scan reports.
- Assess contractions (frequency and duration).
- Monitor progress in labour (examine 2–4 hourly).
- If there is delay in cervical dilatation (progress less than 0.5–1 cm per hour) commence IV oxytocin infusion if primigravida. In a multigravid woman, oxytocin should only be used where poor progress is thought to be due to inadequate contraction frequency (less than 4 in 10 min)
- If there is delay in the 2nd stage, assisted vaginal delivery can be performed using long-handled traction forceps if the presenting part is mento-anterior and at the level of (or below) the ischial spines. The angle of traction is the same as for an occipito anterior position with the head delivering once the chin is below the symphysis-pubis by flexion.
- Ventouse delivery is contraindicated.
- Rotation of head—only mento-anterior position will deliver successfully vaginally. Persistent mento-posterior positions require delivery by CS.
- Head may flex during labour to become a brow (see above).
- Monitor fetal heart rate.
- Fetal blood sampling cannot be performed for heart rate abnormality (deliver by CS).
- Skilled operators may consider the use of rotational forceps if the position is not direct mento-anterior and the head is low in the pelvis.
- CS can be difficult due to the inability to flex the head to assist with delivery.

☠ **Anaesthetic complications on the labour ward**

The majority of anesthetic complications on the labour ward are caused by the method of pain relief used i.e. opiates or local anesthetics. Fortunately serious complications are rare.

Immediate actions
- Initiate immediate life support measures (ABC) if patient has had a cardio-respiratory arrest or is in imminent danger of an arrest.
- If patient has had an arrest—call cardiac arrest team and alert theatres and on-call obstetrician of possible emergency CS.
- If not immediately life-threatening, call anesthetist.
- Stabilize patient's vital signs—pulse, blood pressure, SaO_2.
- Monitor fetus and take any necessary action.
- Start appropriate monitoring to gauge patient's progress.
- Once patient is stable seek causes and start definitive treatment.

Side effects of opiates

Opiates can be administered via intrathecal/epidural/IV/IM routes. All can produce the following side effects.
- Nausea and vomiting
- Pruritus
- Drop in blood pressure
- Decreased conscious level
- Respiratory depression
- Respiratory arrest

Nausea and vomiting
- Very stressful and unpleasant for patient.
- Prolonged vomiting can lead to dehydration.
- Check blood pressure as hypotension can cause nausea and vomiting.
- Treat with antiemetic e.g. metaclopramide 10 mg IV or IM. 6 hourly as required.
- Start IV fluids as rehydration has been shown to be helpful.

Pruritus
- Distressing for patient.
- Initial treatment is with an antihistamine e.g. chlorpheniramine (Piriton™) 10 mg IV or IM.
- If persists call anaesthetist.
- Consider rarer causes
  - adverse blood reaction
  - adverse drug reaction
  - cholestasis—check serum bilirubin

Side effects of local anaesthetics

Usually administered via spinal or epidural route

Accidental IV injection or cumulative toxicity, producing high cerebral and myocardial tissue levels.

- Cerebral irritability leading to seizures
- Cardiac depression from profound negative inotropic action on myocardium—drop in blood pressure
- Major arrhythmias
- Cardiac arrest.

If block spreads too high (usually volume related)

- Hypotension (blocking mid–high sympathetic nerves)
- Bradycardia (blocking T1–T4)
- Respiratory arrest (direct action on respiratory centre)
- Loss of consciousness (direct action on brain stem and higher cerebral function)
- Profound cardiovascular collapse (direct action on brain stem centres).

Hypotension (BP < 80 systolic or >20% drop in systolic pressure)

- Place patient in left lateral position to decrease aortocaval compression.
- Tilt bed head-down or raise legs to increase venous return.
- Give rapid IV bolus of 500 ml fluid.
- Give oxygen via a facemask.
- Monitor fetus.
- If pressure still low give ephedrine 3–6 mg every few min until desired response obtained.
- Consider other causes e.g. intra-abdominal bleeding.
- Continue to monitor patient carefully once resuscitated.

Severe bradycardia

(Heart rate <45/min: often associated with concomitant hypotension.)

- If associated with a procedure e.g. venepuncture or vaginal instrumentation, the cause is likely to be a vasovagal response—stop procedure: check pulse and blood pressure and treat appropriately.
- If hypotensive—treat as outlined above. Place in left lateral position, head down.
- Give oxygen via facemask.
- Ensure good IV access.
- Monitor fetus.
- Arrange for continuous ECG monitoring.
- Give atropine 600 µg IV. Repeat every 30 sec up to a maximum dose of 3 mg.
- Call for anesthetic help.
- If bradycardia persists consider adrenaline IV. Start with 50 µg and repeat dose every 30 sec until heart rate is >60/minute. NB adrenaline can cause severe hypertension and tachycardia.

Seizure
- Most seizures are of short duration.
- The primary aim is to support mother during seizure and prevent self-damage.
- Place patient in coma position (left lateral—head down) to prevent respiratory obstruction and aspiration of gastric contents.
- Ensure good IV access.
- Never place your fingers in patient's mouth.
- Give oxygen via facemask.
- If fit prolonged or recurring give 5 mg diazepam (or diazemuls) IV followed if necessary by a further 5 mg IV.
- Consider if this could be an eclamptic fit? If yes—start magnesium protocol.
- If seizure caused by local anesthetic toxicity, be vigilant for possibility of profound cardiovascular collapse occurring within a few minutes.

Loss of consciousness
- Place patient in coma position (left lateral—head down) to prevent gastric aspiration.
- Clear airway and administer high flow oxygen via facemask.
- Support airway with head tilt and forward jaw thrust.
- Call anaesthetist urgently.
- Monitor patient's oxygen saturation, blood pressure, and pulse in case situation deteriorates further.
- Ensure good IV access.
- Monitor fetus.
- If patient has had an opiate—give naloxone 0.4 mg IV. If limited or no response repeat dosage. NB naloxone has a short half-life and patients can become re-narcotized within 30 min.
- If patient is on magnesium stop infusion and obtain urgent plasma levels.
- Patient must be continuously monitored for the next few hours.

Respiratory arrest
- Regardless of cause this is a medical emergency.
- **Call cardiac arrest team**.
- Feel for carotid or femoral pulse. If no pulse start full CPR immediately.
- If pulse present start respiratory resuscitation immediately: mouth-to-mouth or via self-inflating bag and mask with 100% O_2.
- If able to ventilate easily turn patient into left lateral position, head down to decrease risk of acid aspiration.
- If not able to ventilate in left lateral position—place patient supine with a wedge to decrease aortocaval compression.
- Institute full none invasive monitoring; ECG/SaO_2/non-invasive automatic blood pressure monitoring.
- Ensure good IV access.
- Monitor fetus.
- Alert theatre and obstetric team of possibility of emergency CS.

- If opiates have been given, administer naloxone 0.4 mg IV. Repeat if necessary.
- If on magnesium infusion stop infusion and obtain urgent plasma levels.
- Consider other causes:
  - post seizure
  - cerebral bleed
  - wrong drug administered
- If diagnosis still unsure seek urgent neurological advice.

Cardiac arrest

See ABC of resuscitation in pregnancy, pp. 18–21.

Post-delivery procedures and complications

Kevin Hayes and S. Arulkumaran

Abdul Sultan

Ranee Thakar

Leonie Penna

Kate Farrer

⊕ Retained placenta

Non-delivery of the placenta (partly or wholly) within 30 min of fetal delivery despite adequate attempts to deliver it. This time period is arbitrary and poorly defined. Most would agree placental delivery should be complete within 1 hour.

Retained placenta affects 0.5–3% of women following delivery and is a considerable cause of maternal morbidity and mortality especially in the developing world.

Associations

- Previous retained placenta (commonest)
- Prematurity
- Induction of labour
- Increasing multiparity
- Increasing age
- Known placental abnormality e.g. succenturiate lobe/double placenta
- Placenta praevia
- Previous CS/uterine trauma e.g. multiple curretage (predisposes to morbid adherence—placenta accreta/increta/percreta).

Risks

- Post-partum haemorrhage
- Intrauterine infection and sepsis
- Uterine inversion (if over-zealous traction applied)
- Hysterectomy
- Maternal death.

Prevention

Evidence shows active management of the 3rd stage (oxytocin/ergometrine, cord clamping, controlled cord traction) significantly reduces the risk of PPH, but possibly increases the risk of retained placenta compared to physiological management.

Management

Assess degree of bleeding and haemodynamic status

If actively bleeding or haemodynamically compromised *act quickly*:

- RRR: remedy the cause, replace volume, replace oxygen carrying capacity.
- IV oxytocin infusion (40 iu in 500 ml normal saline).
- Blood for FBC and G&S (crossmatch 2–4 units if Hb < 10 g/dl or active bleeding).
- Catheterize the bladder.
- Judicious attempt at controlled cord traction.
- **Avoid** excessive traction.
- If undelivered after 30 min make plans for manual removal under anaesthesia.
- **Anticipate PPH at all stages.**

Manual removal of placenta (MROP)

- Perform in theatre.
- Adequate anaesthesia (usually epidural/spinal).
- Sterile technique (operator to use gauntlet gloves).
- Prophylactic broad spectrum antibiotic cover (e.g. cefuroxime + metronidazole).
- Use hand to progressively dilate cervix.
- Tocolysis is rarely required unless access to the cavity is manually impossible.
- Manually shear placenta off uterine wall along the plane of cleavage/separation.
- Remove placenta wholemeal if possible and check whether it is complete.
- Re-explore cavity to check if empty.
- Bimanual compression of uterus to reduce inevitable bleeding.
- Repair any perineal or vaginal tears as appropriate.

There is some evidence that administration of oxytocin into the umbilical vein (at least 20 units) may reduce the incidence of need for MROP. This may be particularly worth trying in the developing world where safe MROP may not be easily accessible.

In the event of non-delivery of the placenta

When the placenta is morbidly adherent (placenta accreta/increta/percreta) and does not separate at manual removal or is very difficult then no further attempts should be made to deliver it as there is an increased risk of heavy bleeding and the need for hysterectomy.

Options

If bleeding is minimal and does not continue

- Leave the placenta undisturbed (antibiotic and oxytocic cover).
- Placenta tends to autolyse and separate and get extruded.
- Methotrexate is of questionable use (no reduction in rates of PPH).

If active bleeding

- Bilateral uterine artery embolization.
- Hysterectomy—preferable if the family is complete and no desire for future fertility or the bleeding is causing haemodynamic disturbance.

:☠: **Post-partum haemorrhage (PPH)**

Bleeding (revealed or unrevealed) from the genital tract, after delivery, of more than 500 ml. It occurs in 5–10% of deliveries and is a leading cause of maternal mortality worldwide (>125 000 women die each year). PPH is usually the 3rd or 4th commonest cause of death in the triennial Confidential Enquies into Maternal Death. Estimated blood loss is highly subjective and often underestimated.

Primary PPH—>500 ml from delivery up to 24 hours or blood loss that causes haemodynamic disturbance if it is less than 500 ml (e.g. in an anaemic or underweight mother).

Secondary PPH—>500 ml 24 hours to 6 weeks.

Massive obstetric PPH—loss >1500 ml and is a life-threatening condition— rapid action is required to prevent death.

Risk factors
- Previous PPH
- APH
- Multiple pregnancy/polyhydramnios
- Grand multiparity (≥ para 5)
- Operative delivery especially emergency LSCS.

Anticipation and prevention
- Identify risk factors and plan accordingly (IV access/Hb/G&S or crossmatch in labour).
- Active management of the 3rd stage (prophylactic oxytocics, clamp and cut cord, and controlled cord traction) reduces the risk from approximately 10% to nearer 5%.

Causes (4 T's)
- *Tone*—uterine atony is the commonest cause of PPH by far (80–90%).
- *Trauma*—cervix, vagina, perineum, anus, and rectum. Rarely there is injury into the broad ligament or other organs such as the bladder, uterine rupture, or inversion.
- *Tissue*—retained placenta (wholly or partly).
- *Thrombin*—development of DIC especially in massive haemorrhage, pre-eclampsia, amniotic fluid embolism, or sepsis.

Management (3 R's)
- *Remedy* the cause
- *Replace* volume
- *Replace* oxygen carrying capacity
- Resuscitate the mother—assess pulse, BP
- Lie flat and give oxygen
- Insert 2× 14G IV cannulae
- IV crystalloid (colloid if collapsed)
- Send blood for Hb and cross-match 2–4 units
- Rub up a contraction
- Catheterize the bladder

- Commence IV infusion of oxytocin 40 iu in 500 ml normal saline over 2–3 hours
- Ergometrine 500 µg IM is highly effective
- Misoprostol 800 µg PR is also useful
- If uterine atony persists then carboprost (PGF2α) 250 µg IM or intra-myometrial is also effective (this can be repeated at 15 min intervals up to a maximum of 1 mg).
- Treat the underlying cause—the above aim to resuscitate and treat uterine atony.
- If bleeding persists then quick recourse to EUA in theatre is indicated.
- If bleeding is approaching 1000–1500 ml and is ongoing then senior obstetric, anaesthetic, and haematological attendance is required— **CALL FOR HELP**.
- EUA—the whole genital tract including upper vagina and cervix is inspected for tears, repaired as appropriate, and the uterine cavity is explored manually to exclude placental fragments. Broad spectrum antibiotic cover is needed to cover the bacteraemia (cefuroxime and metronidazole or augmentin IV).
- When there is diffuse bleeding from vaginal lacerations, tight packing of the vagina with gauze can be highly effective.
- If bleeding continues then other measures available are: balloon tamponade (Sengstaken/Bakri balloon) of the uterine cavity with up to 500 ml of warm saline instilled into the intracavity balloon) can lead to instant cessation of bleeding. *Those that do not stop immediately require a laparotomy.*
- Options at laparotomy:
  - Ligation of uterine and utero-ovarian vessels through avascular windows in the broad ligament and mesovarium respectively (reducing uterine perfusion pressures).
  - Ligation of anterior divisions of internal iliac arteries after stripping off the overlying parietal peritoneum (further reducing uterine perfusion pressures).
  - B-lynch or brace suture or vertical compression suture (2–4) to externally tamponade the uterine cavity.
  - Uterine artery embolisation (interventional radiology) is another fertility saving procedure that can successfully reduce bleeding.
  - Hysterectomy is the last resort when bleeding is intractable— subtotal hysterectomy is highly effective, quicker and usually safer than total hysterectomy.

Where women have died the same observations are commonly noted: underestimated loss, inadequate fluid and blood replacement, decision for hysterectomy left too late, lack of timely senior multidisciplinary input.

Blood products

Replacing red cells and coagulation factors to improve oxygen carrying capacity and correct coagulopathy is vital once loss over 1500 ml is reached or sooner if there is haemodynamic compromise or the pre-delivery haemoglobin was low to begin with.

Fully cross-matched whole blood is preferred but group specific non-cross-matched blood may be given if the clinical situation is severe. As a general rule:

- 1 unit of blood equivalent to 1 g/dl of haemoglobin.
- 2 units of fresh frozen plasma (FFP) required for every 5 units of blood cryoprecipitate (rich in factor VIII) and platelets may also be required.
- If bleeding is completely intractable then activated factor VIIa has been successfully used as a last resort.

Expert haematological advice is vital when there is massive haemorrhage and transfusion needs are urgent or coagulopathy becomes apparent.

In the event of massive PPH it is important to have a **labour ward protocol** activated to ensure appropriate multi-disciplinary help is available. Contemporaneous accurate documentation including timings is vital. High dependency unit (HDU) care is also important for aftercare.

After-care (HDU)

- HDU trained midwife/nurse 1:1 care.
- Senior obstetric/anaesthetic/haematological input.
- Monitor lochia, wound, and abdominal signs as appropriate.
- Pulse oximetry (beware of pulmonary oedema and ARDS).
- BP/pulse/temp recording every 15 min.
- CVP monitoring.
- Arterial line may be required on anaesthetic advice.
- Urine output (hourly).

☼ Vaginal and perineal lacerations

More than 85% of women sustain perineal trauma after vaginal delivery and up to two thirds of these women will require suturing. Perineal trauma may occur either spontaneously during vaginal birth or a surgical incision (episiotomy) is intentionally made to enlarge the diameter of the vaginal outlet. It is also possible to have a spontaneous tear in addition to an episiotomy. The episiotomy incision begins at the posterior fourchette and may be mediolateral (incision directed laterally to avoid the anal sphincter) or midline (directed vertically towards but not including the anus). Although the midline episiotomy is associated with less bleeding, less pain, and better healing, it is more likely to extend and involve the anal sphincter. Midline episiotomies are preferred in North America and mediolateral episiotomies are preferred in Europe.

Perineal lacerations are classified as follows:[1]

- First degree: laceration of the vaginal epithelium or perineal skin only.
- Second degree: involvement of the perineal muscles but not the anal sphincter.
- Third degree: disruption of the anal sphincter muscles which should be further subdivided into:
  - 3a: <50% thickness of external sphincter torn.
  - 3b: >50% thickness of external sphincter torn.
  - 3c: internal sphincter also torn.
- Fourth degree: a third degree tear with disruption of the anal epithelium.

It is also possible to get an isolated laceration of the rectal mucosa (buttonhole) without involvement of the anal sphincter.

Aetiology

- Normal vaginal delivery
- Instrumental delivery
- Shoulder dystocia
- Malpresentation and malposition
- Big baby.

Diagnosis

Symptoms

- Bleeding
- Pain.

Signs

- Anaemia or shock may occur if with severe post-partum haemorrhage or haematoma.
- Perineal tears may be associated with involvement of the anal sphincter (third or fourth degree tears).
- Fever may develop if infection develops.

Management

- Manage shock.
- Perform rectal examination to exclude anal sphincter involvement.
- Vaginal examination to establish extent of tear.

- Ensure adequate analgesia (top-up epidural or inject local anaesthetic).
- First degree tears do not need suturing unless associated with bleeding.
- It is recommended that all second degree tears should be sutured unless it is the explicit wish of the woman to the contrary.
- If multiple lacerations are present, each laceration should be repaired individually ensuring anatomical and cosmetic restoration.
- Repair of a second degree tear (including episiotomy) is performed in layers approximating vaginal epithelium, perineal muscles using a continuous, non-locking method and subcuticular suturing of skin. Vicryl Rapide[TM] is associated with less perineal pain and need for suture removal.[1,2] Rectal examination should be performed after repair to check for inadvertent insertion of sutures through the anal epithelium.
- All third and fourth degree tears must be repaired in the operating theatre under regional or general anaesthesia.[3] If torn the anal epithelium is repaired with interrupted 3-0 Vicryl[TM] sutures with the knots tied in the anal canal. The internal anal sphincter is approximated using mattress sutures with 3-0 PDS sutures. The external sphincter can be repaired by the end-to-end or overlap technique using 3-0 PDS sutures. The perineal body should be reconstructed in the same manner as described for second degree tears. All women with third and fourth degree tears should be prescribed antibiotics. Laxatives should be prescribed for 7–14 days. Hospital follow-up should be arranged.

Prevention

- Restrictive rather than liberal use of episiotomy
- Mediolateral rather than midline episiotomy
- Vacuum extraction is preferable to forceps
- Antenatal perineal massage can be beneficial.

References

1. Royal College of Obstetricians and Gynaecologists (2004). Methods and materials used in perineal repair. RCOG Guideline No. 23. London: RCOG Press.
2. Kettle C, Hills RK, Jones P, et al. (2002). Continuous versus interrupted perineal repair with standard or rapidly absorbed sutures after spontaneous vaginal birth: a randomised controlled trial. Lancet, **359**, 2217–23.
3. Thakar R, Sultan AH (2003). Management of obstetric anal sphincter injuries. The Obstetrician and Gynaecologist, **5**, 31–9.

☠ Uterine inversion

Uterine inversion is said to occur when the fundus inverts into the uterine cavity. Incomplete inversion occurs when the fundus, though inverted, does not herniate through the cervix. Complete inversion occurs when the fundus has passed completely through the cervix and lies within the vagina, or more rarely outside the vulva.

The incidence of uterine inversion varies from 1:2000 to 1:50 000 deliveries depending upon the standard of management of the 3rd stage of labour. It is more likely to occur in primiparous patients and when there is a fundal placenta, morbidly adherent placenta, uterine abnormalities and/or short cord.

Aetiology

- In majority of cases it occurs due to mismanagement of the 3rd stage involving fundal pressure and/or cord traction performed before placental separation.
- Too rapid withdrawal of the placenta during manual removal or at CS.
- It may also occur without mismanagement of the 3rd stage when there is a sudden rise in intra-abdominal pressure when the uterus is relaxed e.g. coughing or vomiting.

Diagnosis

Symptoms

- Severe lower abdominal pain
- Bleeding per vagina.

Signs

- Placenta may or may not be *in situ*
- Shock out of proportion to blood loss due to increased vagal tone
- Haemorrhage, present in 94% cases
- Uterine fundus not palpable per abdomen (in incomplete cases there may be a dimple in the fundal area)
- Pelvic examination showing a mass in the vagina or outside the introitus.

Management

- Manage shock.
- Attempt to reposition the uterus. The earlier the repositioning the more likely the success.[1] Delay in replacement of the uterus is associated with formation of a cervical ring and increasing oedema and congestion of the uterus. Do not attempt to remove the placenta if still attached to the uterus. Immediate non-surgical techniques are successful in most cases.

Techniques to replace the uterus

Manual replacement

The technique for replacement of the uterus is to cup the fundus in the palm of the hand, with the fingertips at the junction of the cervix and the corpus, lift the entire uterus out of the pelvis towards the umbilicus. This position is maintained for a few minutes until firm contraction of the uterus occurs. If the placenta is not delivered it is removed manually at this stage. Manual replacement of the uterus is preferable under general anaesthesia as it requires the uterus to be relaxed. Tocolytic drugs e.g. magnesium sulphate, ritodrine, terbutaline may be used to relax the cervical ring to facilitate replacement.[2]

Hydrostatic repositioning (O'Sullivan technique)[3]

Ensure that there are no tears in the vagina, cervix, or uterus. Infuse warm saline into the vagina (via a rubber tube held 1–2 m above the patient) while the vagina is blocked by the assistant. As the vaginal vault is distended with fluid the fornices are ballooned and stretched, pulling on the constricting cervical ring and facilitating spontaneous reduction of the uterus. Alternatively an intravenous giving set can be attached to a silicone Ventouse cup inserted in the vagina, which can produce a better seal.[3]

Surgery

This is attempted if conservative treatment fails. It involves performing a laparotomy and the uterus is repositioned by the following techniques.

- *Huntingtons technique:* Allis forceps are placed within the dimple of the inverted uterus. Gentle traction is applied on the clamps with further placement of forceps on the advancing fundus.
- *Haultains technique:* this involves incising the cervical ring posteriorly with a longitudinal incision. This facilitates enlargement of the constricted cervical ring and replacement of the uterus. The incision is sutured. After repositioning the uterus oxytocics should be administered to prevent recurrence.

Prevention

Avoid mismanagement of 3rd stage. Cord traction should not be applied until signs of placental separation appear, i.e. trickle of blood at introitus, lengthening of the cord, and globular hard contracted uterus on palpation.

References

1. Watson P, Besch N, Bowes WA (1980). Management of acute and subacute puerperal inversion of the uterus. *Obstet Gynecol*, **55**, 12–16.
2. Johnston R, Cox C. Uterine inversion. In: R Johanson, C Cox, K Grady, C Howell (eds). Managing obstetric emergencies and trauma. The MOET course manual pp. 183–4. RCOG Press (2002), London.
3. O'Sullivan J (1945). Acute inversion of the Uterus. *BMJ* **2**, 282–3.

⚙ Vulval/perineal haematoma

A haematoma may occur in the vulval/perineal and vaginal area either immediately following delivery or in the post-partum period. They occur infrequently, with an incidence of between 1:500 to 1:900 pregnancies.

Aetiology
- Frequently related to episiotomy
- Can occur despite delivery with intact perineum (approximately 20%).

Diagnosis
Symptoms
- Pain in the perineal area
- Swelling of the perineal area
- Occasionally may present with shock in spite of no obvious swelling. This can occur when there is a paravaginal haematoma. The classical presentation is pain, restlessness, inability to pass urine, and rectal tenesmus a few hours after delivery.

Signs
- Obvious tender, swelling of the perineal area. Overlying skin may appear purple and glistening.
- Signs of shock depending on the amount and rate of blood loss.

Management
- Management of shock if present.
- Surgical evacuation by incision and drainage if the haematoma is large and expanding. Incision should preferably be made in the vagina to avoid scar formation. Achieve haemostasis. Often no obvious bleeding points are seen. A large vulval haematoma may benefit by leaving a drain or pack in it.
- If small (i.e. <5 cm) and not expanding use ice-packs and pressure dressings.
- Appropriate analgesia.

Prevention
The perineum should be carefully examined after delivery and in the immediate post-partum period.

☠ Obstetric collapse

Causes

Obstetric collapse may occur at any time during pregnancy. Sudden loss of maternal consciousness is potentially the most serious emergency occurring during pregnancy. The differential diagnosis will depend on whether the woman is antenatal, intra-partum or postnatal.

- Non-serious 'collapse' vaso-vagal episode
- Haemorrhagic shock:
  - Obstetric:
    — APH
    — PPH
  - Non-obstetric:
    — aortic dissection
    — hepatic rupture
    — rupture of splenic artery aneurysm
    — rare causes (AV malformations, other aneurysms).
- Uterine inversion
- Cardiogenic shock:
  - myocardial infarction
  - cardiomyopathy
  - cardiac disease
- Adrenal crisis
- Pulmonary embolism
- Septic shock
- Anaphylactic shock
- Amniotic fluid embolism
- Cerebrovascular accident
- Hypoglycaemia
- Drug toxicity.

Management

- Assessment and initial management must occur simultaneously
- Call for help (cardiac arrest team may be required)
- Commence basic life support
- If breathing spontaneously give high-flow oxygen via face mask with reservoir bag in all cases
- If antenatal and >24 weeks gestation use wedge for left lateral tilt
- Insert 2 large bore (16G minimum) intravenous cannula
- Commence monitoring (automated blood pressure/pulse), pulse oximeter, cardiac rhythm monitor)
- Insert urinary catheter.

Investigations

- FBC, U&E, LFTs coagulation screen on all
- G&S
- C-reactive protein and blood cultures (suspected septic shock)
- Fibrinogen and FDPs (possible disseminated intravascular coagulation)
- Blood gases
- 12-lead ECG

- Request portable chest X-ray
- Abdominal ultrasound.

Making a diagnosis
- Rapid review of antenatal notes for risk factors
- Obtain history of events immediately prior to collapse
- Some diagnoses such as obstetric haemorrhage are obvious others will require investigation
- Examine woman to assess cardiac and respiratory status (JVP, heart auscultation and full respiratory assessment)
- Examine woman for specific signs (abdominal tenderness, neurology).

Diagnosis-specific management
Peri-mortem Caesarean delivery
- Request CS set immediately in all cases of antenatal cardiopulmonary arrest (>24 weeks gestation).
- If advanced life support with effective tilt is unsuccessful after 5 min, commence to assist in maternal resuscitation.
- Crash call senior paediatrician to assess baby (delivery is to assist resuscitation not to save baby).
- Request sterile gloves, scalpel and blade.
- Shaving, swabbing, and draping the abdomen is unnecessary in this circumstance.
- Vertical or horizontal (Cohen's) abdominal incision are acceptable, whichever the operator feels will be quickest.
- Vertical uterine incision saves time by avoiding need to reflect bladder.

Amniotic fluid embolism
Consider diagnosis in any woman collapsing intra-partum or immediately post-delivery. Amniotic fluid embolism may occur in women delivered by CS. Recent rupture of membranes is not essential for diagnosis. Initial presentation is of massive right-sided heart failure. Severe left-sided heart failure and disseminated intra-vascular coagulation may follow in women who survive the initial presentation
  Management principles:
- Ventilation with 100% O_2.
- Maintenance of cardiac output with crystalloid and inotrophs.
- Admission to intensive care unit for invasive monitoring.
- Aggressive treatment of coagulopathy (platelets, fresh frozen plasma, and cyoprecipitate).
- Requires urgent delivery if antenatal and successful resuscitation (assisted vaginal delivery if possible or CS).
- Anticipate possible massive post-partum haemorrhage and manage promptly.

Septic shock
Consider the possibility in any woman with previous diagnosis of infection, prolonged rupture of membranes, immuno-compromise, or post-CS.
- Consider possibility of appendicitis.
  Management principles:
- Administer crystalloid and inotrophs.

- Culture for source of infection prior to commencing broad spectrum IV antibiotics in appropriate doses.
- If antenatal and resuscitation successful deliver only if signs of fetal compromise.

Adrenal crisis

Consider in any woman taking high dose steroids.
  Management principles:
- Crystaloid fluid replacement
- Fluids to replace electrolyte imbalance (hyponatraemia, hyperkalaemia occur with Addisionian crisis)
- 50% dexrose if hypoglycaemia (glucocorticoid deficiency)
- Give hydrocortisone 100 mg IV.
- If antenatal and resuscitation successful deliver only if there are signs of fetal compromise.

Anaphylaxis

Consider possibility of latex allergy or if new drug was recently administered.
  Management principles:
- Give 0.5 ml of adrenaline 1 in 10 000 (may require repeat and infusion 0.1 mg/min if blood pressure remains low).
- Crystalloid volume expansion.
- Antihistamines (chlorpheniramine 10–20 mg IV) infusion.
- Maintain BP and adequate renal perfusion judged by urinary output—dopamine 2–10 µg/kg/min is useful.
- Hydrocortisone 200 mg IV.
- Inhaled salbutamol if bronchospasm (or IV 250 µg).
- If antenatal and resuscitation successful deliver only if there are signs of fetal compromise.
- Full allergy testing on recovery and avoid stimulus in future.

Magnesium toxicity

Magnesium sulphate toxicity is very rare with standard doses but consider possibility of drug error or in women with impaired renal function.
  Management principles:
- Stop magnesium infusion and withhold until levels available.
- Give 10 ml of 10% calcium gluconate IV over 2 min.
- Send blood for magnesium levels.
- If antenatal consider expediting delivery (Caesarean or assisted vaginal delivery) as pre-eclampsia is now further complicated.

☠ Resuscitation of the newborn

1–10% of newborns require resuscitation at delivery.[1] The need for resuscitation is often unpredictable thus it is essential that all personnel who attend deliveries are able provide initial neonatal resuscitation.

Preparation

Personnel

A Paediatrician should be present for the following deliveries:

- Emergency CS
- Instrumental deliveries
- Meconium stained liquor
- Fetal distress
- Cord prolapse
- Breech deliveries
- Multiple births
- Preterm deliveries <37 weeks gestation
- Infants of diabetic mothers
- Congenital abnormalities (antenatal diagnosis)

Equipment

Ideally prepare and check prior to the delivery:

- Resuscitaire with air/oxygen mix—turned on
- Heater—turned on
- Suction—checked with selection of catheters sizes
- Clock—set to zero
- Stethoscope
- Laryngoscope—2 sizes, good light source
- Face masks—size 00, 0/1
- Pressure delivery system, usually T-piece set to 25–30 cm H_2O
- Resuscitation/Ambu bag—500 ml
- Emergency sterile equipment e.g. for umbilical vein and IV access
- Drugs—see p. 164

Assessment and action

3 basic steps of resuscitation are:

Airway
Breathing
Circulation

See NLS algorithm for summary (Fig. 6.1)

1. At delivery:
   - If concerned CALL FOR HELP
   - Start clock
   - Dry and wrap baby on resuscitaire
   - Assess:
     —breathing—quality and quantity
     —heart rate—assess at apex with stethoscope or palpate at base of cord; assess as slow <60, adequate >100
     —colour—centrally pink, pale or cyanosed; peripheral cyanosis is common and unimportant if baby otherwise well
     —tone—active, reduced or floppy.

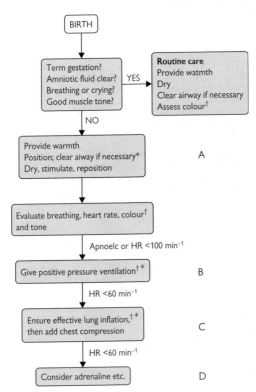

BIRTH

Term gestation?
Amniotic fluid clear?
Breathing or crying?
Good muscle tone?

YES

Routine care
Provide watmth
Dry
Clear airway if necessary
Assess colour†

NO

Provide warmth
Position; clear aiway if necessary*
Dry, stimulate, reposition   A

Evaluate breathing, heart rate, colour†
and tone

Apnoelc or HR <100 min⁻¹

Give positive pressure ventilation†*   B

HR <60 min⁻¹

Ensure effective lung inflation,†*
then add chest compression   C

HR <60 min⁻¹

Consider adrenaline etc.   D

* Tracheal intubation may be considered at several steps

† Consider supplemental oxygen at any stage if cyanosis persists

Fig. 6.1 Newborn Life Support. Reproduced with permission of Resuscitation Council (UK)

2. Obviously healthy: good respiratory effort and good heart rate, pink and active → dry and give to mother.
3. Poor respiratory effort or primary apnoea, good heart rate →
   • Open airway by positioning head in neutral position (see Fig. 6.2)
   • Stimulate
   • Gentle suction at 8–10 kPa (60–75 mmHg) negative pressure only if obvious secretions; over zealous suctioning can cause vagal arrest and delay respiration
   • Facial oxygen may help
   If no response proceed as below.
4. Poor respiratory effort or apnoea, slow heart rate, cyanosis, floppy → CALL FOR HELP if not already done so.

Airway
• Open airway by positioning head in neutral position (see Fig. 6.2)
• Facial IPPV via face mask and T-piece or Ambu bag
• Administer 5 effective inflation or rescue breaths at 30 cm H_2O for 2–3 seconds for term baby
• Effective inflation indicated by good chest movement

If no chest movement **Reassess** and consider
• Check head in neutral position (see Fig. 6.2)
• Jaw thrust—open airway by positioning fingers behind angle of jaw and push jaw forward (see Fig. 6.2)
• Shoulder elevation—elevating baby's shoulders by 1–2 cm with a towel placed under them can help to open the airway
• 2-man manoeuvre with one operator holding face mask with 2 hands whilst second operator provides IPPV; this technique is good for large babies
• Guedel airway
• Whether airway not blocked with secretions, meconium or blood; observe under direct vision and, if indicated, suction under direct vision with 8–10 size catheter at 8–12 kPa (60–100 mmHg) negative pressure
• Higher inflation pressure

Breathing
• If despite 5 effective inflation breaths there is no spontaneous respiration continue with one sec ventilation breaths at 30–60/min; use appropriate pressure to give effective chest movement, this is usually lower than inflation breaths e.g. 20–25 cm H_2O for term baby
• Proceed to endotracheal intubation only if you are experienced. Most babies can be ventilated for the initial resuscitation with facemask IPPV as long as the chest movement is good
Reassess after 30 sec of effective ventilation breaths.

(a)

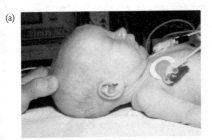

(b)

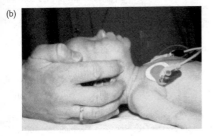

Fig. 6.2 (a) Neutral position. Newborn babies have a prominent occiput and thus adopt a flexed head posture when prone. (b) The neutral position is neither extended or flexed; jaw thrust has also been applied here. Figs. 6.2a and b are reproduced with permission of: Resuscitation Council (UK).

Circulation
Do not proceed to cardiac compressions until effective ventilation with adequate chest movement achieved.

The commonest cause of slow heart rate is ineffective lung inflation. If heart rate remains slow despite adequate ventilation:
- Provide chest compressions by:
  - Encircling chest with both hands, placing thumbs over lower third sternum and fingers around back of chest, or
  - 2 finger technique—place index and middle finger over lower third sternum
- Depress lower third sternum by depth of 1/3 or 2–3 cm for term baby
- Provide 3 compressions to one effective ventilation at ratio of 3:1 or 30 cycles/min or 120 events/min

Reassess after 30 sec

Drugs

If heart rate remains slow, ≤60 bpm, despite effective lung inflations and cardiac compressions, gain IV access via cut down and catheterization of umbilical vein or peripheral venous access. Administer:

Adrenaline (epinephrine)

- 0.1 ml/kg 1:10 000 IV stat followed by 2–3 ml–saline flush
- Continue CPR
- Repeat adrenaline every 3 min
- Try 0.3 ml/kg if 3rd dose necessary
- 1st dose can be given via ETT if no IV access but higher doses of 0.3–1.0 ml/kg 1:10 000 might be needed by this route

Sodium bicarbonate

- Acidosis decreases adrenaline binding at cardiac receptors thus consider IV $NaHCO_3$ if resuscitation prolonged
- Administer 2–4 ml/kg 4.2% $NaHCO_3$ followed by 2–3 ml saline flush

Dextrose

2–3 ml/kg 10% dextrose followed by 2–3 ml saline flush.

Volume

If evidence of hypovolaemia, especially acute blood loss, give 10–20 ml 0.9% saline or O Rh negative blood.

Naloxone

If mother had intrapartum opiates and the baby remains apnoeic but otherwise well despite appropriate resuscitation—administer 100–200 mcg/kg naloxone IM.
NB: Do not give naloxone if mother opiate dependent

Born dead/fresh still-birth

Apnoeic, no HR, white, floppy → CALL FOR HELP if not already done so
- Initiate full ABC resuscitation as above
- If no response after 10 min then it is appropriate to consider stopping resuscitation
- Ideally a senior paediatrician needs to be involved in this decision
- Transfer baby to NICU if resuscitation successful

Post resuscitation

- Cord gas: arterial cord pH and base deficit should be measured and documented in all cases where there has been fetal distress or neonatal resuscitation
- Documentation: needs to be full, logical and clear with a legible signature

Special considerations

1. Temperature
   - Term babies: Wrap and warm baby to maintain normal temperature. Clinical studies assessing the effect of mild hypothermia on neurodevelopmental outcome for term asphyxiated babies are in progress. Already completed studies indicate no significant benefit of selective head cooling[2] and some promising benefit of total body cooling[3]. No significant adverse effects have been reported. Whilst

further evidence is evaluated treatment with hypothermia is currently only available in the UK in centres participating in randomized controlled trials. Overheating is linked to adverse outcome and should be avoided.[4]

- Preterm babies: hypothermia increases adverse outcomes[5] and exacerbates acidosis, hypoxia and RDS. Many centres are applying occlusive wraps or delivering preterm babies ≤30 weeks into plastic bags.[6]

2. Premature babies ≤35 weeks

If possible anticipate delivery, allowing time for senior staff to be present and to communicate with parents outlining the prognosis and discussing the parents wishes.

ABC assessment and action should proceed as for term babies with the following precautions:

- Temperature—see above
- Lower pressure is usually required for inflation breaths e.g. 20–25 cm H_2O; once FRC and effective chest movement is established, the pressure should be reduced to maintain adequate, not overenthusiastic chest movement—try 15–20 cm H_2O
- Babies with severe RDS may need higher pressure for inflation breaths e.g. 30 cm H_2O
- Babies requiring intubation <30 weeks should receive surfactant as soon as possible by a skilled operator.[7] This is often administered in the labour ward
- Do not give adrenaline under 27 weeks
- CPAP: many premature babies, including some extremely preterm babies may not need intubation in the labour ward. There is some evidence that CPAP, applied with the correct expertise may be feasible and effective if commenced at birth.[8] Further assessment of CPAP at resuscitation is awaited.

3. Extremely premature babies 23–24 weeks—at the margins of viability

- <23 weeks
  —resuscitation should not be attempted
  —paediatrician should not attend delivery
- 23^{+0}–23^{+6} weeks
  —anticipate delivery to allow senior staff to attend and appropriate communication
  —if baby has spontaneous respiration and HR >60 resuscitation with ET intubation may be initiated; if the baby does not improve and the HR remains low at 10 min then further resuscitation should be withheld. Do not give adrenaline
  —if the baby is in poor condition with poor/absent respiration, low/absent HR, often with extensive bruising, it may be kinder not to attempt resuscitation and to give the baby to the mother
- ≥24 weeks
  —these babies should be resuscitated but the same principles apply
  —commence ABC resuscitation as described above
  —stop resuscitation if poor response at 10 min
  —do not give adrenaline

4. Meconium stained liquor
   Perineal suction and routine tracheal intubation for suction have been shown to be of no benefit.[9,10]
   Assessment and action:
   - Good respiratory effort and pink
     —dry and give to mother
     —observe as inpatient for 24 hr
   - Poor respiratory effort
     —**CALL FOR HELP**
     —assess airway under direct vision; if meconium present then suction under direct vision with a large-bore catheter e.g. size 10 or above, at 8–12 kPa (60–100 mmHg) until airway patent. Withdraw catheter as suction applied
     —repeat if meconium still in airway
     —once meconium removed if respiration ineffective then further appropriate ABC management should be initiated
     —trainees are sometimes incorrectly concerned with how long they should suction for before commencing facial IPPV; once airway patency has been established, with suction under direct vision, then inflation breaths should be given with further ABC resuscitation as necessary
     —babies requiring extensive resuscitation need admission to NICU
     —babies who are well post resuscitation should stay with their mother but must be reviewed at 1 hour of age and at regular intervals for 24 hr. Any concerns, particularly tachypnoea with respiratory rate >60 bpm, should be reported to a paediatrician immediately

5. Air v O_2 for resuscitation
   Recent evidence highlights concerns of increased adverse outcome in babies resuscitated with 100% O_2 compared to those resuscitated with air alone.[11] The safest O_2 concentration to use for resuscitation has not been established and it is certainly possible to achieve successful resuscitation with air alone. Whilst further evidence to support appropriate O_2 concentration is awaited a safe, sensible approach includes:
   - Use of resuscitaires which supply air/O_2 mixtures
   - Monitor of O_2 saturation levels during resuscitation
   - Initial use of low O_2 concentration e.g. air–30% and observe effect. If, despite effective ABC management, the baby remains blue then further O_2 should be given.

Poor response to resuscitation
Consider DOPE:
- **D**isplaced tube e.g. in oesophagus or right bronchus
- **O**bstructed tube
- **P**neumothorax—transilluminate or observe for hyperinflation of affected side
- **E**quipment failure:
  - are air or O_2 supplies depleted or disconnected?
  - is pressure setting on T-piece too low or malfunctioning?
  other causes:
  - maternal opiates (see Naloxone administration)
  - congenital diaphragmatic hernia—scaphoid abdomen

- severe asphxia—review history
- severe anaemia—review history and check Hct or PCV (beware: values may be high if recent haemorrhage)

Further reading

1. Resuscitation Council (2001). Resuscitation at Birth Newborn Life Support Course Manual. Resuscitation Council, UK.
2. Resuscitation Council (UK). Newborn Life Support. In: Resuscitation Guidelines 2005 Resuscitation Council 2005 (UK).

References

1. Palme-Kilander C (1992). Methods of resuscitation in low-Apgar-score newborn infants—a national survey. *Acta Paediatr*, **81**, 737–44.
2. Gluckman P, Wyatt J, Azzopardi D, *et al.* (2005). Selective head cooling with mild systemic hypothermia after neonatal encephalopathy: multicentre randomised trial. *Lancet* **365**, 663–70.
3. Shankaran S, Laptook A, Ehrenkranz R, *et al.* (2005). Whole-body hypothermia for neonates with hypoxic-ischemic encephalopathy. *NEJM*, **353**, 1574–84.
4. Petrova A, Demissie K, Rhoads G, Smulian J, Marcella S, Ananth C (2001). Association of maternal fever during labor with neonatal and infant morbidity and mortality. *Obstet Gynecol*, **98**, 20–7.
5. Acolet D, Elbourne D, McIntosh N, *et al.* (2005). Project 27/28: inquiry into quality of neonatal care and its effect on the survival of infants who were born at 27 and 28 weeks in England, Wales, and Northern Ireland. *Pediatrics*, **116**, 1457–65.
6. Vohra S, Roberts R, Zhang B, Janes M, Schmidt B (2004). Heat Loss Prevention (HeLP) in the delivery room: A randomized controlled trial of polyethylene occlusive skin wrapping in very preterm infants. *J Ped*, **145**, 750–3.
7. BAPM Guidelines for RDS, Resuscitation (DRAFT) (2005). BAPM London.
8. Finer N, Carlo W, Duara S, *et al.* (2004). Delivery room continuous positive airway pressure/positive end-expiratory pressure in extremely low birth weight infants: a feasibility trial. *Pediatrics*, **114**, 651–7.
9. Vain N, Szyld E, Prudent L, Wiswell T, Aguilar A, Vivas N (2004). Oropharyngeal and nasopharyngeal suctioning of meconium-stained neonates before delivery of their shoulders: multicentre, randomised controlled trial. *Lancet 14*, **364**, 597–602.
10. Wiswell T, Gannon C, Jacob J, *et al.* (2000). Delivery room management of the apparently vigorous meconium-stained neonate: results of the multicenter, international collaborative trial. *Pediatrics*, **105**, 1–7.
11. Tan A, Schulze A, O'Donnell CP, Davis PG. Air versus oxygen for resuscitation of infants at birth. *Cochrane Database Syst Rev.* **2005**: CD002273

Chapter 7

Miscellaneous topics in obstetrics

Kevin Hayes and S. Arulkumaran
Emergency cerclage *170*

Olujimi Jibodu
Trauma in pregnancy *172*
Transfer and transport of pregnant women *178*

Austin Ugwumadu
Post-partum infections *182*

**Rukma Bhattacharya and
Sambit Mukhopadhyay**
Pharmacotherapeutics in obstetrics *186*

☼ Emergency cerclage

This is performed acutely to prevent a likely or inevitable 2nd trimester miscarriage when the underlying diagnosis is deemed to be cervical incompetence. Cervical incompetence however, is poorly defined and there is no clear diagnostic test. The diagnosis may be clinical, where there is often a history of previous mid-trimester loss or repeated cervical instrumentation or ultrasonographic with cervical shortening and/or funneling.

Indications

- Painless dilatation of the cervix between 12–24 weeks. The procedure is most effective if dilatation is ≤ 4 cm though the procedure has been carried out up to full dilatation. This can be diagnosed by speculum or transvaginal (TVS) ultrasound examination.
- Transvaginal cervical length < 20 mm with dilatation is associated with mid trimester miscarriage and premature delivery.
- Bulging amniotic membranes (hourglass effect) are commonly seen at the same time.
- The procedure may be performed in the presence of minimally painful uterine contractions as these are considered a secondary phenomenon after initial dilatation.

Contraindications

- Fetal death
- Ruptured membranes
- Strong uterine contractions
- Heavy PV bleeding
- Clinical or haematological evidence of acute infection (systemically unwell, offensive vaginal discharge, pyrexia > 37.5°C, unexplained maternal or fetal tachycardia, increased WCC, increased CRP)
- If cervical dilatation is >4 cm success is less likely.

The woman and partner need to understand that the prognosis for the pregnancy is very poor and that there is no clear evidence of benefit for the use of emergency cerclage. Evidence suggests some prolongation of pregnancy but no overall effect on perinatal mortality—numbers are small and there is heterogeneity in cases, diagnostic criteria, and cerclage technique. Live birth rates have been reported between 40–60% in retrospective case series. The procedure therefore is offered on the understanding that the possible benefits of the procedure outweigh the risks in an attempt to prevent a clinically inevitable miscarriage.

Procedure

1. Fully informed consent including procedure related risks including failure of the procedure (resulting in miscarriage), bleeding, rupture of membranes, introduction of infection and cervical damage.
2. Regional anaesthesia required (rarely GA).
3. Aseptic surgical technique.
4. Lithotomy position.
5. Preferably 2 assistants to retract vaginal walls.

6. Anterior and posterior lip of the cervix is grasped with a sponge-holding forceps to facilitate the cerclage.
7. When the cervix is more than 4 cm dilated, more sponge forceps may be needed to define the cervix and to help insert the suture.
8. Insertion of a purse-string, non-absorbable, Mersilene McDonald suture at 3, 6, 9, and 12 o'clock on the cervix tied anteriorly. The aim is for suture placement at the level of the internal os. Sometimes practically, 'as high as safely possible' on the cervix has to suffice. Bulging membranes can be effectively reduced by inserting a 30 ml Foley catheter between the cervix and the membranes. Once inserted the 30 ml balloon can be filled with up to 50 ml saline thus lifting the membranes out of the way of the suture.
9. A small moist swab on holder is also useful.
10. Percutaneous amnioreduction prior to suturing has been described to reduce bulging membranes with varied success and cannot be recommended.
11. Antibiotics (clindamycin, or cephradine and metronidazole) are commonly used to cover the procedure and for 5–7 days after. This is of no proven benefit to pregnancy outcome.
12. Tocolysis and being nursed supine with elevation of the legs are also commonly practiced with no evidence of benefit.
13. Transabdominal approach has been used for emergency cerclage but again is of no proven benefit and has higher operative morbidity.

Removal of suture

- 37–38 weeks gestation for successful ongoing pregnancies
- Painful uterine contractions
- Evidence of infection.

☤ Trauma in pregnancy

Trauma is common in pregnancy, majority (>90%) are minor. Adverse pregnancy outcome occurs in up to 4% of minor injuries and fetal loss is in the range of 40% in critical maternal injury.

Causes

Road traffic accidents (RTA), falls, domestic accidental and non-accidental injury, assault, penetrating trauma.

Anatomic and physiologic effects of pregnancy

• Blood volume increases by up to 50% in pregnancy.
• Up to 30% of blood volume may be lost before pulse and blood pressure change.
• Uterine perfusion may be compromised while maternal pulse and blood pressure are still maintained.
• Reduced venous return in supine position.
• Blood loss into uterus/abdomen may be concealed.
• Uterine size and position render it more prone to trauma.
• Fetus may be more immediately affected than mother.
• Delayed gastric emptying increases risk of vomiting and aspiration.

Approach to management

For major trauma, immediate resuscitation is often carried out by the para-medic/trauma team. The woman is then transferred to an appropriate secondary or tertiary centre, depending on nature, extent, and severity of injuries.

In most countries, women carry a copy of their maternity records, which provides a synopsis of the antenatal care with results of investigations.

Initial assessment is as for any trauma patient, maternal resuscitation is the first priority. Advanced trauma and life support (ATLS) principles of resuscitation allow uniform and smoother management. Fetal assessment should follow achieving stabilisation of maternal condition. Early involvement of obstetricians by trauma team and vice versa is crucial.

Primary survey

This reveals immediately life-threatening problems.

A = airway control using chin lift, suction, or oropharyngeal airway as appropriate. Avoid moving neck/tilting head if possibility of neck injury. Establish cervical spine control/apply cervical collar/sandbags. Call anaesthetist early for airway problems.

B = breathing/ventilation: give O_2 once airway control is achieved. Pulse oximetry valuable in monitoring.

C = circulation: CPR if cardiac arrest; control of haemostasis/IV lines using large bore cannulae and aggressive infusions. Warm infusions when large volumes used. Blood group usually known or recorded in hand-held notes so cross-match is rapid. Central venous access may be crucial when peripheral veins are inaccessible, e.g. in severe shock or extensive burns (although siting a central line is more hazardous). Once neck injury is excluded, left lateral position or 15 degree left tilt will relieve IVC pressure and improve venous return.

D = disability (neurological assessment): with orientation and responsiveness, pupillary reaction, motor response, and Glasgow coma scale.

Levels are <u>a</u>lert, <u>v</u>oice responsive, <u>p</u>ain responsive, <u>u</u>nconscious (note that unresponsiveness may be due to hypovolaemia).

E = exposure: (to allow full/physical examination).

Primary survey—resuscitation phase

Problems identified in the primary survey that need immediate attention are dealt with as they are identified.

Fetal viability and well-being are assessed after primary survey/resuscitation. Depending on maternal and fetal status, delivery may be indicated. Determine gestation (clinical estimation if history is not available), lie, presentation, and listen for fetal heart. Ultrasonographic assessment may be done when patient is stabilized. Electronic fetal heart rate monitoring may be considered if appropriate.

Secondary survey

Secondary survey identifies and deals with problems that are not immediately life threatening. It is performed when the maternal condition is stable and involves more detailed assessment and investigations. Maternal health remains the overriding priority and X-rays, CT, and MRI scans are safe in pregnancy. However, only tests that will influence management need be done. Reference ranges that apply to pregnancy should be used in interpreting test results, e.g. Hb of 10–11 g/dl is not unusual in pregnancy. This is due to plasma volume expansion exceeding red cell mass expansion, resulting in a physiological anaemia.

Adequate exposure should be done without compromising warmth, to allow complete physical evaluation. Up to 50% of the mortality in severe trauma patients is due to head injuries so a neurological assessment is necessary. All neck injuries should be considered life-threatening and receive prompt and adequate attention.

When a chest tube is indicated, it should be placed 1–2 intercostal spaces higher than would otherwise have been indicated. This allows for the elevation of the diaphragm that occurs in pregnancy.

▶ Return to ABC if any deterioration in status.

▶▶ Unless trauma is primarily obstetric, obstetric evaluation is part of the secondary survey. Unstable neck or spine injuries and femoral fractures contra-indicate pelvic examination as the positioning will worsen these conditions.

Definitive care phase

This is dictated by the type of injury and its severity.

General measures

Urinary catheter allows examination of urine for haematuria as a sign of pelvic trauma and urine output as an indicator of renal perfusion. Urine output of 30 ml/hour indicates good renal perfusion.

Kleihauer test is useful in determining feto-maternal haemorrhage and dose of Rh globulin for Rhesus negative women. To avoid undue delay, 250 U SC up to 20 weeks gestation and 500 U after 20 weeks can be given while awaiting test result.

Check tetanus immunization status if indicated by nature of injuries.

Additional treatment options

Emergency (perimortem) CS may be necessary if mother has cardiac arrest and CPR unsuccessful for 5 min, despite left lateral tilt. ▶▶ Formal surgical preparation is not necessary and haemostasis is not an issue. ▶ Maternal resuscitation should continue through the CS. The fetus is relatively resilient to maternal hypoxia for short periods but the 1° aim of the perimortem CS is to facilitate maternal resuscitation.

Other indications for CS in pregnant trauma patients are:

• Inadequate exposure during laparotomy for other abdominal trauma
• Unstable pelvic or lumbosacral fracture with patient in labour
• Uterine rupture
• Placental abruption.

Laparotomy may be necessary for abdominal injury. Haemorrhage may be diagnosed by focused abdominal sonography for trauma (FAST).

DVT risk ↑ in pregnancy. Hypovolaemia and immobilization increase the risk. Prophylaxis with heparin should be considered once risk of haemorrhage is controlled.

▶ Consider the possibility of drug or alcohol intake depending on the nature of trauma.

Persistent shock in trauma patients

Life-threatening problems in the chest

• Airway obstruction
• Tension pneumothorax
• Open pneumothorax
• Massive haemothorax
• Flail chest
• Cardiac tamponade.

Other systemic problems

• Neurogenic shock
• Uncorrected hypothermia
• Hypoxia
• Acid–base/electrolyte imbalances.

Pregnancy specific traumas

• Amniotic fluid embolism
• Placental abruption
• Uterine rupture
• Eclampsia and its complications.

Seat belts

Maternal death is more likely from ejection from the moving vehicle and is the commonest cause of fetal death in RTA. Seat belts are protective at all stages of pregnancy as unrestrained passengers are likely to have impact injuries with the interior of the vehicle or be ejected, with potentially severe injuries to head, face, chest, abdomen, and pelvis. Maternal mortality risk when the passenger is ejected from a moving vehicle is about 30% versus 5% when restrained.

The three-point lap and shoulder restraint is best, reducing the likelihood of moderate to critical injury by 50% and fatal injury by 45%. It should be worn correctly, with the shoulder belt passing between the breasts and over the top of the fundus and the lap belt passing below the uterus. Injuries sustained with this belt in place include sternum, clavicle, and rib fractures. Hollow viscus and lumbar spine injuries may occur with lap-only belts and clavicle, cervical spine, rib, and liver injuries with shoulder-only belts. Airbags may cause abrasions to face and chest.

Blunt trauma

This is the commonest type of trauma in pregnancy, the main cause being from RTA. Most injuries are relatively minor and even major injuries are more likely to be non-obstetric. Obstetric complications include preterm labour, fetomaternal haemorrhage (FMH), placental abruption, and uterine rupture.

Blunt trauma also results from falls and physical assault. Recurrent presentation with minor blunt trauma should raise the suspicion of domestic violence as this is known to either start or worsen in pregnancy.

Major peritoneal haemorrhage is more likely in advanced pregnancy because of the large blood supply to the uterus. Haemorrhage may develop slowly and repeated assessment is necessary to detect any deterioration in physical condition.

Placental abruption is the commonest cause of fetal death when the mother has sustained blunt injury. There may not be obvious abdominal injury to raise the suspicion of fetal trauma. Signs include vaginal bleeding, tense and tender uterus, fetal heart rate abnormalities, and maternal haemodynamic conditions worse than would be explained by the obvious injuries or blood loss.

In addition to the priority management of the mother's trauma, obstetric management will depend on the duration of gestation, maternal condition, and the degree of fetal compromise if any. A particular complication to exclude and monitor is DIC.

▶ Corticosteroids should be given to improve fetal lung maturity when gestation is less than 34 weeks and delivery can be delayed.

▶ Vaginal delivery is not excluded in the presence of placental abruption. CS should be avoided if maternal condition is stable and there is DIC or a dead fetus.

Preterm labour

It may be difficult to determine if uterine activity after blunt trauma is due to labour or placental abruption. If preterm and placental abruption is considered unlikely, tocolysis may be used, especially if the mother is being transferred between units or circumstances dictate that it is of benefit to improve fetal lung maturity with corticosteroids. Note that some of the side-effects of tocolytic agents e.g. β-mimetics and nifedipine are similar to signs of blood loss.

Uterine rupture

This is uncommon as uterine muscle elasticity reduces the risk of rupture. ↑risk of rupture with maternal pelvic fracture and scarred uterus from previous CS. Fetal mortality risk is close to 100% with traumatic uterine rupture. Absence of fetal heart sounds, easily palpable fetal parts, shock disproportionate with injury are leading signs. Management includes obstetric and surgical laparotomy at which other visceral injury should be excluded.

Fetomaternal haemorrhage (FMH)

Risk of FMH is up to 30%, vs. 8% in pregnancies with no reported trauma. Nature and severity of maternal trauma do not correlate well with FMH. Sequelae include Rhesus isoimmunization in Rh negative women carrying an Rh positive fetus, fetal anaemia, and fetal demise. Kleihauer testing is used to quantify the volume of FMH and dose of Rh globulin that needs to be given to the Rh negative mother.

Penetrating injury

This is uncommon and may be due to stab or gunshot. In early pregnancy, the uterus is pelvic and pattern of injury is similar to that in non-pregnant. In late pregnancy, the uterus is abdominal and large, making fetal injury more likely. The high perinatal mortality rates associated may be due directly to the injury or the complications of resultant premature delivery. The maternal viscera are displaced and relatively less prone to penetrating injuries. When bowel is affected, multiple penetrating wounds are more likely, due to the compression of more bowel in a smaller area. Laparotomy should be undertaken by joint obstetric and surgical team but if uterus is not involved, delivery may not be necessary.

Burns

May be due to flame, scalds, chemical or electrical burns. Most are minor, resulting from domestic accidents. More severe burns may occur from house fires and accidents with hot or flammable liquids or gases. Severity and extent are described in terms of depth (full or partial thickness) and the total body surface area affected. The 'rule of nines' used to estimate area of burns underestimates the increased surface area of the abdomen.

Classification

- Minor: partial thickness <10% of surface area.
- Major: partial or full thickness burns >10%.
- Moderate: 10–19%.
- Severe: 20–39%.
- Critical 40% or more.

Obstetric complications of major burns include: premature labour and delivery and fetal death. Early delivery may be considered to optimize maternal management. Corticosteroids should be considered if gestation is less than 34 weeks and the maternal condition permits the necessary delay. CS if necessary can be performed through burnt skin without additional morbidity.

Maternal mortality risk

- <40% burns: <3% mortality
- 40–59% burns: 50% mortality
- 60% burns: 90–100% mortality.

Fetal mortality

- 20% maternal burns: fetal mortality unlikely
- 20–39% maternal burns: 10–27% fetal mortality
- 40–59% maternal burns: 45–53% fetal mortality
- 60% burns: up to 100% fetal mortality.

▶ If the fetus is of viable age, delivery is indicated if maternal burns are 50% or greater. With major burns, fetal loss tends to be within 5 days of burns.

Management
Women with minor burns need analgesia and appropriate wound dressing. Initial management of women with major burns is similar to all trauma victims. Subsequent care should involve burns team. Factors to be considered include: surface area involved, depth of burns, body parts affected (facial burns imply higher risk of inhalation injury), inhalation, associated injuries.

Inhalation injury from burns
Concurrent inhalation injuries may affect the prognosis. Immediate or delayed airway obstruction may occur so secure and maintain airway early.

▶ Suspect inhalational injury when:
• Fire in enclosed space
• Voice alteration
• Facial burns
• Coughing up dark sputum
• Respiratory distress.

If inhalational injury suspected, check arterial blood gases (ABG) for carbon monoxide (CO). CO crosses the placenta and achieves higher concentrations (10–15x maternal levels) in the fetus. The fetus needs a longer time than the mother to eliminate CO.

Signs of CO poisoning:
• 10–20% CO: palpitations, headaches
• 20–40% CO: dizziness, confusion, agitation, incoordination
• >40% CO: dyspnoea, coma and death.

Management
• 10–20% CO blood levels: treat with 100% O_2 by face mask. Time to restore fetal levels to normal may be 5x that of mother, so extended therapy is needed.
• 20% CO or more/neurological features irrespective of CO level: treat with hyperbaric O_2.

Electrocution
Electrocution is very rare and is predominantly from domestic accidents. Cardiac arrest is the commonest cause of maternal death from electrical injury. Cardiac arrhythmias may be delayed so continuous cardiac monitoring is prudent.

Injuries are varied, including those due to falls from the shock. Early consultation and joint management with a trauma team with appropriate experience is advisable.

The fetus is very vulnerable to electrocution and mortality risk is high if it is in the path of the current e.g. hand–foot path. Fetal outcome therefore does not correlate well with the degree of maternal injury. When the fetus survives the initial shock, continuous monitoring is indicated. If at term, delivery should be considered as the fetal effect of the trauma is difficult to assess. If not delivered, regular monitoring including growth scans are advised.

⑦ Transfer and transport of pregnant women

It is sometimes necessary to transfer pregnant women for:
- Failure to progress during labour at home
- Failure to progress during labour at peripheral or midwifery unit to obstetric unit
- Transfer to specialist unit for investigation or treatment of maternal medical illness
- In-utero transfer of fetus for neonatal intensive care. This is the commonest indication for maternal transfer between hospitals.

Assessment for transfer

Transfer of any ill patient from one location to another is often necessary to provide better care than available at the starting point. The risks of staying must outweigh the risks of transfer so it is important that the right patient is transferred at the right time, by the right personnel to the right place using the right mode of transport.

Transportation is usually initiated by the clinicians already caring for the patient or paramedics if from the site of an accident. If transfer is being carried out by an external team, appropriate briefing on arrival on the patient's condition is necessary before the team departs with the patient.

Some maternal conditions are not suitable for transfer e.g.
- Fulminating pre-eclampsia
- Ongoing haemorrhage
- Imminent delivery.

In these circumstances, delivery may have to be undertaken in the referring unit and the baby transferred for neonatal intensive care or the mother transferred if indication is maternal illness. It is important to avoid separating mother and baby so obstetric and neonatal units need to communicate early to ensure appropriate arrangements are made for both.

Controlling the transfer

The transfer team should have clear lines of duty set out, if not already existing. This should include leadership, tasks to be performed during the transfer, and who performs them. A named person e.g. the transferring consultant will have overall responsibility for the transfer.

Communication

Decisions and responsibility for transfers must be taken at consultant level. The clinicians initiating a transfer should agree with the receiving unit that a transfer is appropriate and the facilities to undertake the appropriate care are available. These include:
- Antenatal bed (liaise with obstetric team)
- Appropriate intrapartum facilities (liaise with obstetric team)
- Appropriate expertise (liaise with obstetric and paediatric surgery teams)

- Neonatal intensive care cot (liaise with neonatology team).

The need to transfer should then be discussed with the patient and/or relatives. Appropriate ambulance transportation is then arranged. Ambulance control will determine the type of ambulance provided based on:

- Patient's clinical condition
- Urgency of transfer
- Needs and potential problems during transportation
- Distance to travel
- Number of accompanying persons.

▶ It is vital that full and accurate information be provided. A copy of medical records or summary should be provided for the transfer. This will be handed to the receiving unit.

Transfer categories depend on clinical urgency and severity of patient's illness. Categories are:

- Intensive
- Time critical
- Ill and unstable
- Ill and stable
- Unwell
- Well.

Preparation for transfer

The patient's condition must be stabilized before transfer so that the rigours of travel can be withstood. Inadequate resuscitation before transfer is likely to cause deterioration in patient's condition during the trip. Appropriate personnel, IV fluids, drugs, oxygen and equipment, including neonatal respiratory support must be available in the ambulance.

The patient should be secured to the trolley which is in turn secured to the ambulance. Wedging is important to prevent aortocaval compression. All lines, drains, monitoring and drug administration equipment also need to be secured. Accompanying persons should be securely seated and restrained. It may however become necessary during a transfer for procedures to be carried out (e.g. delivery of a baby). It may be necessary for the ambulance to remain stationary for this and resume the trip afterwards.

Arrangements for the return trip for the accompanying staff and relatives must be confirmed before setting out on the trip. The ambulance is not obliged to return them.

Apart from the ambulance crew, the patient must be accompanied by a midwife if the pregnancy is over 34 weeks and/or there is little or no risk of delivery in transit. Other accompanying personnel will depend on the indication for transfer and potential problems anticipated. If there is a risk of delivery, especially if preterm, it may be more appropriate for that to be undertaken at the referring unit and the neonate transferred (ex-utero) instead.

Tocolysis is usually used to reduce the risk of delivery during in-utero transfers. Corticosteroids are administered concurrently to promote fetal lung maturity if the fetus is less than 34 weeks.

Mode of transportation is determined by:

- Nature of illness

- Urgency of transfer
- Geographical factors e.g. accessibility by road
- Distance to travel
- Traffic conditions on the route.

Most transfers are over relatively short distances and road ambulances are most appropriate. Air ambulances are more expensive but more appropriate if the distance is long or road access is restricted or unfavourable.

Seek expert advice if long distance air ambulance is considered necessary. Effects of the plane's microclimate need to be considered and air flight may be contra-indicated.

If the patient being transferred is a trauma victim, continuous assessment and maintenance of resuscitation principles (ABC) is necessary.

Handover

At the destination, the patient should be directly handed over to a senior member of the receiving unit. Medical records and details of monitoring or events during the transfer should be passed on.

☼ Post-partum infections

Background
Puerperal sepsis is a polymicrobial condition, which occurs in a small minority of women, suggesting that the pathogenesis involves more than just a source of potentially pathogenic bacteria. As pregnancy progresses, there is a 10-fold increase in the population of protective *Lactobacillus* species and a progressive decline in the number of potentially pathogenic anaerobes (*Prevotella bivus, Bacteroides* species, peptococci, peptostreptococci) and *E. coli,* a possible adaptation of the genital tract flora designed to protect the fetus from exposure to harmful bacteria at the time of birth. By the third post-partum day, and regardless of the mode of delivery, the numbers of anaerobic organisms rise again to levels higher than in the antenatal period. This latter rise, believed to be due to the withdrawal of trophic support from the genital tract, and the presence of lochia and necrotic decidua sets the scene for post-partum infections.

Endometritis
Endometritis is the commonest puerperal infection and usually presents within 5 days of delivery.

Risk factors
- CS (27% versus 1.2% in women who had vaginal delivery)
- Multiple vaginal examinations during labour
- Prolonged rupture of membranes
- Use and duration of internal monitoring devices
- Prolonged labour
- Group B streptococcal colonisation
- Anaemia, diabetes mellitus, obesity.

Diagnosis
Criteria for diagnosis include fever, ± chills and rigors, uterine tenderness, ± abdominal pains, purulent or foul smelling lochia, leucocytosis, and exclusion of another focus of infection. There may be tachycardia. Localizing signs may be absent if the infection is due to group A or B streptococcus.

Obtain cervical and vaginal samples for culture.

Treatment
If febrile and unwell—IV broad-spectrum antibiotics with anaerobic cover for example cephalosporin or clindamycin and gentamycin.

Septic pelvic thrombophlebitis
This is thought to be due to bacterial injury to the pelvic (ovarian) venous endothelium. The diagnosis should be considered in any patient with a persistent temperature despite appropriate antibiotic therapy and prior soft tissue pelvic infection.

Clinical features
- Persistent fevers may be the only presentation
- Progressively worsening abdominal pain usually right > left
- Nausea, vomiting, or abdominal distension may be present

- Bowel sounds may be normoactive or absent
- Tachycardia
- Tachypnoea and respiratory distress if pulmonary embolus has occurred
- The thrombosed ovarian vein (usually right) may be palpable as an abdominal or adnexal mass.

Investigations
- Ultrasound scan
- CT scan.

Treatment
- Broad-spectrum antibiotic therapy
- Anticoagulation with heparin was a traditional adjunct to therapy but this is no longer recommended.
- Surgical ligation/excision of the affected vein is reserved for patients with acute abdomen or not responding to medical therapy.

Urinary tract infection

This is a common cause of post-partum pyrexia and is usually caused by *E. coli* although enterococci, group B streptococci and other Gram-negative aerobic bacilli may occasionally be responsible. Symptoms include dysuria, frequency, nocturia, fever, and backache. Physical examination may reveal tenderness in the renal angles. A clean catch specimen of urine for culture is helpful in diagnosis. Sterile pyuria may reflect bladder inflammation from trauma during labour and delivery.

Risk factors
- Physiologic hydroureter of pregnancy
- Asymptomatic bacteriuria
- Intra-partum catheterization.

Treatment

Parenteral cephalosporin and gentamycin initially until urine cultures and antibiotic sensitivities become available.

Mastitis and breast abscess

Staphylococcus aureus is the main causative agent of sporadic, epidemic, and endemic mastitis. Fever, malaise, and breast pain and tenderness are the usual presenting features. Breast abscess may develop in untreated cases.

Treatment

A penicillinase-resistant penicillin such as flucloxacillin or erythromycin should be administered. Other measures include breast support, ice packs, and analgesics. Breastfeeding should continue unless abscess develops.

Wound and episiotomy infections

Around 5–15% of CS wounds become infected depending on the definition of wound infection used. The presence of erythema, induration, pain, and fluid exudate are suggestive signs. If the wound breaks down, debridement and secondary closure is now recommended instead of the traditional approach of debridment and dressing, and allowing healing by secondary intention. Clinicians should maintain a high index of suspicion in order to recognise life-threatening wound complications such as necrotizing fasciitis, clostridial myonecrosis (gas gangrene) and non-clostridial bacterial synergistic gangrene (Meleney gangrene).

A simple episiotomy infection usually presents with localized erythema, oedema and exudate, which are limited to the surrounding skin and subcutaneous tissue. If the findings are more extensive, a deeper infection may be present. The wound should be opened, explored, drained, and debrided, and appropriate antibiotics administered. Most of these will heal by granulation but if perineal muscles or anal sphincter is involved, the wound should be re-sutured once the infection settles down, say in about 5–10 days. The patient should avoid sexual intercourse and have sitz baths 3–4 times daily.

⑦ **Pharmacotherapeutics in obstetrics**

Analgesics

Simple analgesics like paracetamol or combination of paracetamol and codeine phosphate are often used in pregnancy for non-specific pain in the abdomen, UTI, headache, and any muscle pain, after ruling out serious pathology. Opiates are commonly used for pain relief in labour.

Paracetamol (acetaminophen)

Side effects and dosage are not different from non pregnant patients. Pharmacokinetics also does not differ significantly. It should be used with caution in patients with hepatic and renal impairment.

Pethidine (meperidine)

Pharmacology

It is an opioid analgesic, predominantly μ receptor agonist. Its main action is on the CNS and the neural elements in the bowel.

Use

Moderate to severe pain, obstetric analgesia, perioperative analgesia.

Dose

- For pain relief in labour, administer 50–100 mg by SC or IM route.
- Can be repeated 1–3 hr later if necessary.
- Maximum dose 400 mg in 24 hr.
- Better avoided within 3 hr of delivery.
- Postoperative pain—SC or IM 25–100 mg every 2–3 hr.

Pharmacokinetics

Onset of analgesic effect is within 10 min after SC or IM injection. Though it is absorbed by all routes of administration, rate of absorption after IM injection may be erratic. Peak plasma concentration occurs at about 45 min. It is metabolized chiefly in liver, with a half-life of 3 hr. It crosses the placenta and can cause neonatal respiratory depression.

Side effects

- Nausea, vomiting, constipation
- Drowsiness
- Larger dose can cause respiratory depression and hypotension
- Ureteric and biliary spasm
- Bradycardia, tachycardia, palpitation
- Hallucination, mood change
- Pruritus
- Convulsion
- Dependence.

Drug interaction

- MAO inhibitors cause CNS excitation or depression (upto 2 weeks after discontinuation).
- Chlorpromazine and tricyclic antidepressants increase the CNS depressant effects.
- Selegiline can cause hyperpyrexia and CNS toxicity.
- Cimetidine inhibits metabolism of pethidine.
- Ritonavir (antiviral) increases the plasma concentration.

Contraindication
- Acute respiratory depression
- Acute alcoholism
- Raised intracranial pressure
- Head injury
- Pheochromocytoma (risk of pressure response to release of histamine)
- Severe renal impairment.

Antibiotics

The following antibiotics are considered safe in pregnancy:
- Penicillins
- Co-amoxiclav
- Cephalosporins
- Erythromycin
- Clindamycin.

Definition of food and drug administration classification

FDA classification	Definition
Category A	Well-controlled studies in human show no felt risk
Category B	Animal studies show no risk, but human studies inadequate *or* Animal studies show some risk, but not supported by human studies
Category C	Animal studies show risk, but human studies are inadequate or lacking *or* No studies in humans and animals
Category D	Definite fetal abnormalities in human studies, but potential benefits may outweigh the risks
Category X	Contraindicated in pregnancy, fetal abnormalities in animals or humans, risks outweighs the benefits

FDA classification of drugs used in nausea and vomiting in pregnancy

Generic names	FDA classes
Pyridoxine	A
Cyclizine	B
Diphenhydramine	B
Metochlopramide	B
Prochlorperazine	B
Ondansetron	C
Corticosteroids	C

Antibiotics are used in obstetrics for various infections e.g. urinary tract infection (UTI), respiratory tract infection, and also for prophylaxis e.g. ruptured membranes, cardiac valve abnormality (during labour), prevention of group B streptococcal infection in baby during labour etc.

Prevention of Group B Streptococcus infection in the baby is an important indication of antibiotic treatment. Group B Streptococcal infection can cause fatal neonatal septicaemia. Penicillins are commonly used as prophylaxis in labour.

For women in labour, the recommended doses of penicillin G are 3 g (or 5 mega units) IV initially and then 1.5 g (or 2.5 mega units) at 4-hourly intervals until delivery. For women who are allergic to penicillin, clindamycin should be prescribed, the recommended dose is 900 mg IV every 8 hours until delivery.

To optimise the efficacy of antibiotic prophylaxis, the first dose should be given at least 2 hours prior to delivery.

Elective Caesarean sections

Women undergoing planned CS in the absence of labour or membrane rupture do not require GBS antibiotic prophylaxis, irrespective of their GBS status, since the risk of neonatal GBS disease is extremely low.

Other situations

- Antibiotic prophylaxis for GBS is unnecessary for women with preterm rupture of the membranes—unless they are in established labour.
- If chorioamnionitis is suspected, broad spectrum antibiotic therapy, including an agent active against GBS should replace GBS-specific antibiotic prophylaxis.
- Pharmacokinetics of some common antibiotics is discussed on pp. 282–290.

Antiemetics

Nausea and vomiting in pregnancy is a common experience affecting 50–90 per cent of all pregnant women. Hyperemesis gravidarum is the most severe manifestation of the spectrum of nausea and vomiting of pregnancy. It requires hospitalization for IV fluid therapy and antiemetics. A variety of antiemetics are used in pregnancy. None of them have FDA category A approval but fortunately teratogenic effect on human foetuses has not been reported with any of the commonly used antiemetics.

The commonly used antiemetics are

Antihistamines

Cyclizine 50 mg 8 hourly, oral, IM or IV.

Phenothiazines

Prochlorperazine (stemetil) is a phenothiazine group of drug. It is a dopamine antagonist and acts centrally by blocking the chemoreceptor trigger zone. The dose used in severe vomiting is 12.5 mg 8 hourly by IM inj. or 5 mg rectal suppository. In milder cases oral tablet 5 mg tds.

Extrapyramidal symptoms and drowsiness are the main side effects

Promotility agents
Metoclopramide

It has both central as well as peripheral antidopeminergic effects. It can be given orally (10 mg tds) or parenterally. The known side effects are extrapyramidal effects, hyperprolactinemia, and drowsiness.

Anticonvulsives

Magnesium sulphate

Pharmacology
Magnesium sulphate has been shown to be very effective in the management of eclampsia, a life threatening obstetric emergency. It prevents recurrent seizures. The exact mechanism of action of magnesium sulphate is not known.

Dosage
Regimens for management of eclampsia vary in different hospitals, but usually the initial IV dosage is 4 gm (over 5–10 min), followed by infusion at a rate of 1 gm/hr for 24 hr after last seizure. Additional IV bolus of 2 gm can be given in case of recurrence of seizure. Same regimens are used for seizure prophylaxis in severe pre-eclampsia.

Monitoring
Monitoring for clinical signs for overdose is essential. Urine output (100 ml in last 4 hr), respiratory rate (> 16/min), and patellar reflexes (lost in overdose) are checked regularly.

Calcium gluconate (10%–10 ml) can be used for management of magnesium toxicity.

Side effects
Serious side effects are due to toxicity. These are arrhythmia, drowsiness, confusion, loss of tendon reflex and respiratory paralysis.

Drug interaction
Profound hypotension has been seen with nifedipine and intravenous magnesium sulphate in preeclampsia. Parenteral magnesium enhances the effect of non depolarising muscle relaxant.

Diazepam
It is a benzodiazepine; acts by enhancing the GABA mediated synaptic inhibition. Regular use is avoided in pregnancy due to risk of neonatal withdrawal symptoms, but can be used for seizure control (e.g. status epilepticus). It was used in the past to treat eclamptic convulsions. However, magnesium sulphate being proved to be more effective it is no longer favoured now.

Antihypertensives
The aim of treating hypertension in acute obstetric emergencies like severe pre-eclampsia and eclampsia is primarily to prevent serious maternal complications.

Hydralazine or labetalol infusion is preferred. Sometimes nifedipine is used sublingually to achieve a quick control of severe hypertension. Methyldopa, takes longer to control blood pressure; hence it is not the drug of choice in cases of emergency.

Hydralazine

Pharmacology
It is a vasodilator and acts by direct relaxation of arteriolar smooth muscles. The decrease in blood pressure is associated with a selective decrease in vascular resistance in coronary, cerebral, renal, and placental circulations.

Dosage
- Can be used orally but in emergencies IV route is preferred.
- The usual dose is administered as a slow IV 5–10 mg (diluted with 10 ml normal saline). This may be repeated after 20–30 min.
- Infusion 200–300 µg/min, with a maintenance dose of 50–150 µg/min is used in most units.

Side effects
- Flushing, palpitation, tachycardia, headache, fetal heart rate abnormalities due to reduction in utero placental circulation.
- SLE like syndrome.
- Abnormal liver function, jaundice.
- Pyridoxine responsive polyneuropathy.
- Angina pectoris.

Drug interaction
- Anaesthetics, analgesics, antidepressants, alcohol, anxiolytics, betablockers, muscle relaxants, nitrates all increase the hypotensive effect.
- Corticosteroids decrease the hypotensive effect.

Labetalol
Pharmacology
It is a combined $\alpha 1$ and β receptor antagonist. It lowers blood pressure by reducing vascular resistance. Cardiac output at rest is not reduced.

Dosage
- Oral: 100 mg twice daily, can be increased to 800 mg bd. If dose is higher, should be divided into 3–4 doses. Maximum dose 2.4 gm daily.
- IV injection: 50 mg over 1 min, repeated after 5 min. Max dose 200 mg.
- IV infusion: 2 mg/min until a satisfactory response is seen.
- In acute hypertensive crisis in pregnancy a dose of 20 mg/hr may be required.

Side effects
- Postural hypotension
- Headache, tiredness
- Rashes
- Liver damage.

Contraindication
- History of obstructive airways disease
- AV block
- Severe peripheral arterial disease
- Phaeochromocytoma.

Nifedipine
It is a calcium channel blocker and relaxes vascular smooth muscle and dilates coronary and peripheral arteries.

Dosage
Different preparations have different dosages, but usual initial dose is 10 mg twice daily orally.

Side effects
- Headache, palpitation
- Tachycardia
- Gravitational oedema, rash.

Contraindications
- Cardiogenic shock, congestive cardiac failure
- Advanced aortic stenosis
- Porphyria.

Methyldopa
Pharmacology
It is a centrally-acting antihypertensive which acts via an active metabolite. It is not used in cases of emergencies, but for long-term control of blood pressure.

Dosage
Oral—250 mg tds gradually increased to a max dose of 3 gm daily.

Side effects
- Gastrointestinal disturbances, dry mouth
- Sedation, headache, dizziness, depression
- Hepatotoxicity is an uncommon but serious toxic effect
- Haemolytic anaemia, bone marrow depression.

Contraindication
- Depression
- Active hepatitis
- Phaeochromocytoma
- Porphyria.

Anticoagulants

Anticoagulants are used in pregnancy for prophylactic as well as therapeutic reasons. Prophylactic use is during prolonged bed rest or postoperative period in high-risk cases. Therapeutic use is during pulmonary embolism or deep vein thrombosis. They are also used throughout pregnancy if there is higher risk of DVT or PE due to personal or family history.

Low molecular weight heparins (enoxaparin, tinzaparin)
Pharmacology
They are as effective as the unfractionated heparin. They have longer duration of action and are given once daily in the SC route.

The standard prophylactive regime does not need monitoring.

Dosage
Enoxaparin
- Prophylaxis in moderate risk surgical patients 20 mg 2 hr before surgery and 20 mg every 24 hr.
- In high risk patients 40 mg 12 hr before surgery and 40 mg every 24 hr.
- Therapeutic dose is 1.5 mg/kg every 24 hr.

Tinzaparin
Prophylaxis 3500 units 2 hr before surgery then 3500 units every 24 hr.
Therapeutic dose is 175 units/kg once a day.

Side effects
- Haemorrhage
- Thrombocytopenia
- Hyperkalaemia
- Hypersensitivity.

Drug interactions
Cautious use with NSAID and aspirin.

Contraindication
- Haemophilia and other haemorrhagic disorders
- Thrombocytopenia
- Peptic ulcer, recent cerebral haemorrhage
- Severe hypertension
- Hypersensitivity
- Cautious use during spinal or epidural anaesthesia due to risk of spinal haematoma.

Tocolytics
They are used in cases of preterm labour. Different drugs are used in different hospitals. The followings are the commonly used drugs.

Atosiban
Pharmacology
This is a new drug, which acts against the oxytocin receptors. It is licensed for inhibition of uncomplicated preterm labour between 24 and 34 weeks gestation.

Dosage
Initially 6.75 mg over 1 min by IV injection, then 18 mg/hr for 3 hr, followed by 6 mg/hr for up to 45 hours by infusion. Maximum duration of treatment is 48 hr.

Side effects
Nausea, vomiting, tachycardia, hypotension, headache, dizziness, hot flushes, hyperglycemia.

Contraindication
- Intrauterine infection
- Intrauterine fetal death
- Placenta praevia, abruption
- Abnormal fetal heart rate
- Blood loss needs to be monitored after delivery.

Ritodrine
Pharmacology
This is a selective β2 adrenergic agonist used as a uterine relaxant.

Dosage
IV infusion—initially 50 μg/min, gradually increase by 50 μg/min every 10 min until contractions stop or maternal heart rate is 140 bpm. To be continued 12–48 hr after contractions stop. Maximum rate 350 μg/min.

Side effects
- Tachycardia, palpitation
- Hypotension (left lateral position during the infusion may minimize the risk)
- Pulmonary oedema
- Chest pain or tightness.

Drug interactions
Corticosteroids increase risk of hypokalaemia if high doses of both the drugs are given.

Contraindications
- Cardiac disease
- Intrauterine infection
- Intrauterine fetal death
- APH, placenta praevia.

Nifedipine
Though its use as an antihypertensive is becoming less popular, this drug is being preferred over ritodrine as a uterine muscle relaxant. The green top guideline published by the Royal College of Obstetricians and Gynaecologists has included this drug amongst the tocolytics. However this is not licensed in the UK to be used as a tocolytic and the responsibility lies with the prescribing doctor. The dose used in the largest trial is 10 mg every 15 min for the first hour and then 60–160 mg/day (slow release tablet) depending on uterine activity. However, there is no consensus about the appropriate regimen.

Uterine stimulants
They are used to stimulate or increase uterine contractions. The main uses are induction of labour, augmentation of labour, prevention or treatment of post-partum haemorrhage, management of retained placenta.

Oxytocin (Syntocinon)
Pharmacology
It is a neurohypophyseal hormone, a cyclic nonapeptide. It stimulates both the frequency and the amplitude of uterine contractions. These effects are dependant on oestrogen and the immature uterus is resistant to these effects.

Use
Induction and augmentation of labour. Prophylaxis and treatment of post-partum haemorrhage.

Dosage
30 international units of oxytocin in 500 ml of normal saline will give 1 milliunit per minute if run at 1 ml per hr. Maximum recommended dose is 20 milliunits per min. Infusion is commenced at 2 milliunits per min and escalated at 2 milliunits per min every 30 min until contractions lasting 40 sec recur 4–5 times in every 10 min. The dosage schedule is

indicated in the following table:

Concentration of oxytocin

- 2–16 mu/min is physiological range
- 5–10 mu/min initiates uterine activity comparable to early labour
- 10–15 mu/min generates uterine activity similar to late 1st stage of labour
- 20–25 mu/min produces activity similar to 2nd stage of labour

---

In severe post-partum haemorrhage IV infusion 5–20 U in 500 ml of fluid at a rate sufficient to control uterine atony. (Usually every hospital has a protocol outlining the rate of infusion in cases of post-partum haemorrhage.)

Side effects

- Uterine hyperstimulation leading to fetal distress
- Water intoxication and hyponatraemia associated with high doses with large infusion of electrolyte free fluid
- Nausea, vomiting.

Drug interactions

- Inhalational anaesthetics reduce oxytocic effect
- Prostaglandins have uterotonic effect.

Contraindications

- Mechanical obstruction to delivery
- Fetal distress
- Severe cardiovascular disease.

Ergometrine

Pharmacology

This is an ergot alkaloid and has a very powerful uterotonic action. After a proper dose there is forceful and prolonged uterine contraction and the resting tone is increased and a sustained contracture can occur. This is very effective in controlling atonic uterine bleeding.

Use

Post-partum bleeding, bleeding after miscarriage.

Dosage

500 µg IM injection.

Side effects

- Nausea, vomiting, headache, dizziness
- Transient hypertension
- Abdominal pain, chest pain.

Drug interactions

Risk of ergotism with erythromycin.

Contraindication

- Severe hypertension, eclampsia
- Induction of labour, 1st, and 2nd stage of labour
- Vascular disease
- Severe hepatic and renal impairment
- Severe cardiac disease
- Impaired pulmonary function.

Syntometrine

It is a combination of ergotamine maleate 500 µg and oxytocin 5 U/ml. It is administered by IM injection after delivery of the shoulders to facilitate the separation of the placenta and to reduce blood loss.

Carboprost

Pharmacology

Prostaglandin F2α, produced in the uterus and is a luteolytic hormone in some subprimate species. Its main use is to control bleeding in atonic post-partum haemorrhage where uterus has failed to respond to ergometrine and oxytocin.

Dosage

250 µg deep IM injection, to be repeated if necessary after 15 min. Maximum dose is 2 mg (8 doses).

Side effects

- Nausea vomiting, diarrhoea
- Hyperthermia and flushing
- Less frequently raised blood pressure and dyspnoea and pulmonary oedema.

Contraindications

Cardiac, renal, pulmonary, and hepatic disease.

Further Reading

1. Goodman and Gilman's The Pharmacological Basis of Therapeutics by Hardman J.G., Limbird L.E and Gilman A.G. 10th Edition, August 2001.
2. Tocolytic Drugs for Women in Preterm Labour, October 2002, (Guideline No 1B). Published by Royal College of Obstetricians and Gynaecologists.
3. Antenatal Corticosteroids to Prevent Respiratory Distress Syndrome, February 2004, (Guideline No 7) Published by Royal College of Obstetricians and Gynaecologists.
4. British National Formulary, March 2005, Published by British Medical Association.

Gynaecology

Abnormal menses and bleeding

Sandeep Mane

ⓘ **Heavy menses**

Menorrhagia is defined as heavy regular bleeding in excess of 80 ml. It is a subjective disorder reflecting a change in the patient's perception of, or inability to cope with, the heaviness of the menstrual flow.

Causes

Pelvic

- Organic causes are fibroids, endometriosis, pelvic inflammatory disease, IUCD
- Dysfunctional uterine bleeding. Ovulatory or anovulatory.

Systemic

- Coagulation abnormalities
- Thyroid disorder.

Symptoms

Heavy menstrual loss

It is vital to obtain a detailed history of the menstrual cycles. This includes the length of the cycle and the flow of bleeding. Passage of clots and flooding forcing the patient to use double protection suggests heavy bleeding.

Tiredness, weakness, or easy fatiguability

Anaemia resulting from excessive blood loss leads to tiredness and fatiguability.

Associated symptoms

- Excessive pelvic pain during the cycle suggests uterine cramps resulting from heavy bleeding.
- Premenstrual pain may indicate endometriosis or adenomyosis.
- Dyspareunia may be caused by endometriosis or pelvic inflammatory disease.
- Offensive vaginal discharge may be present in pelvic infections.
- The influence of the above symptoms on the patients lifestyle, such as absence from work and their sex life, help in determining the severity of the symptoms.

Other relevant history

- It is important to obtain detailed past gynaecological history including information about contraception and smear history.
- Information about past pregnancies helps to understand the fertility status and also a recent obstetric event could present with heavy periods.
- Past medical history is important to know of any pre-existing bleeding tendencies and use of anticoagulant medications.
- Weight gain, constipation, and hair loss suggest thyroid disorder.
- Past surgical history may influence the treatment. Suspicion of intra-abdominal adhesions due to past infections or surgery may make vaginal surgery unsafe.

Signs
General examination
This is performed to look for tachycardia, hypotension, and pallor. In addition, signs of hypothyroidism and evidence of bruises or gum bleeding suggestive of clotting disorder may be seen.

Abdominal examination
This is performed to look for any tenderness or masses arising from the pelvis.
- Tenderness may suggest endometriosis or pelvic infection.
- Large fibroids, endometriotic cysts, and tumours could present as abdominal masses.

Speculum examination
It is essential to look for any local cervical or vaginal lesions. It may reveal a cervical polyp or fibroid. It would also be helpful to assess the severity of the blood loss.

Staining of inner aspects of the thighs or legs is suggestive of heavy loss. It is useful to observe a sanitary towel if available. Pad check is one useful way to estimate the blood loss during the hospital stay.

Bimanual examination
This helps to know the uterine size, shape, tenderness, and mobility.
- Enlarged uterus may be present in fibroids and adenomyosis.
- Restricted mobility is present in endometriosis and pelvic infections.
- Tenderness may be a sign of adenomyosis.
- Cervical excitation is a feature of acute adnexal pathology such as pelvic infection.

Investigations
- FBC is performed to look for anaemia. Increased white cell count could suggest pelvic infection.
- Hormonal profile including seum FSH, LH, and testosterone may be required if polycystic ovarian disease is suspected clinically.
- TFTs are done if symptoms and signs are suggestive of thyroid disease.
- Coagulation tests are done if clinically indicated.
- In cases of severe bleeding, one would have to G&S or even cross-match blood.
- Transvaginal ultrasound scan helps to detect any uterine pathology or endometrial abnormality. Endometrial thickness of <8 mm is reassuring in premenopausal women. Endometrial thickness >5 mm in postmenopausal age group warrants further investigations. This could be either endometrial biopsy, or hysteroscopy and D&C.
- Endometrial biopsy must be obtained if possibility of underlying malignancy exists. The risk factors in history include: age >40 years, diabetes, hypertension, obesity, nulliparity, and family history of colon cancer.
- Hysteroscopic evaluation of the uterine cavity can be performed in the outpatient settings ± anaesthesia, or as an inpatient operation. In spite of a normal-looking cavity, endometrial biopsy is essential.
- D&C is a blind procedure and is likely to miss intrauterine pathology and should not be used by itself.

Treatment

1. *Medical*

Hormonal

- Progesterone from day 5 to 26 in a cyclical manner. Progestogens administered from day 15 or 19 to day 26 of the cycle offer no advantage over other medical therapies such as danazol, tranexamic acid, NSAIDs, and the IUS in the treatment of menorrhagia in women with ovulatory cycles. Cyclical progesterone for 21 days of the cycle results in a significant reduction in menstrual blood loss. This treatment is less acceptable than intrauterine levonorgestrel to most women. This regimen may have some role in the short term treatment of menorrhagia.
- Danazol has been found to be an effective treatment for heavy menstrual bleeding compared to other medical treatments. Unfortunately, the androgenic side effects are unacceptable to many women.
- Combined oral contraceptive pills—useful in young women with anovulatory cycles. Combined pills help in regularizing the cycles and also control the flow of bleeding. In addition, contraceptive needs are also covered.

Non-hormonal

- First line of treatment would be tranexamic acid, which is a antifibrinolytic. The gastrointestinal side effects are well-tolerated. It reduces the blood loss by 50%. Antifibrinolytic therapy causes a greater reduction in objective measurements of heavy menstrual bleeding when compared to placebo or other medical therapies (NSAIDs and oral luteal phase progestagens). Any dose-related side-effects can be reduced by limiting the use during the first 3 to 4 days of the period. There is a significant improvement in flooding and sex life after tranexamic acid therapy when compared with oral luteal phase progestogens.
- Prostaglandin synthetase inhibitors—mefenamic acid is also very effective and safe treatment. It reduces the blood loss by 30–40% in 75% of the patients. NSAIDs reduce heavy bleeding when compared with placebo but are less effective than either tranexamic acid or danazol. However, adverse events are more severe with danazol therapy. In the limited number of small studies suitable for evaluation, no significant difference in efficacy was demonstrated between NSAIDs and other medical treatments such as oral luteal phase progestogen, OCC, or IUS.
- Mirena coil insertion—the levonorgestrel-releasing intrauterine device (LNG IUS) is more effective than cyclical norethisterone (21 days) as a treatment for heavy menstrual bleeding. Women with an LNG IUS are more satisfied and willing to continue with treatment but experience more side-effects such as intermenstrual bleeding and breast tenderness. The LNG IUS results in a smaller mean reduction in menstrual blood loss than transcervical resection of the endometrium (TCRE) and women are not as likely to become amenorrhoeic, but there is no difference in the rate of satisfaction with treatment. Women with an LNG IUS experience more progestogenic side effects compared to women having TCRE for treatment of their heavy menstrual bleeding, but there is no difference in their perceived quality of life.

2. Surgical

Surgery reduces menstrual bleeding at one year more than medical treatments, but LNG IUS appears equally beneficial in improving quality of life and may control bleeding as effectively as conservative surgery over the long-term. Oral medication suits a minority of women long-term.

Conservative surgery

- Endometrial ablation techniques give similar, but lower satisfaction rates compared to hysterectomy. These methods have been proven to be relatively safe for symptom control with a quicker postoperative recovery and hospital stay. Endometrial thinning prior to hysteroscopic surgery in the early proliferative phase of the menstrual cycle for menorrhagia improves both the operating conditions for the surgeon and short term post-operative outcome. Gonadotrophin-releasing hormone analogues for 2 months before the planned surgery produce slightly more consistent endometrial thinning than danazol, though both agents produce satisfactory results.
- Endometrial destruction offers an alternative to hysterectomy as a surgical treatment for heavy menstrual bleeding. Both procedures are effective and acceptable to most patients. The cost of endometrial destruction is significantly lower than hysterectomy but since retreatment is often necessary the cost difference narrows over time.
- There is a rapid development of a number of new methods of endometrial destruction. Most of these are performed blind and are technically easier than hysteroscopy-based methods. Overall, the existing evidence suggests success rates and complication profile of newer techniques of ablation compares favourably with TCRE, although technical difficulties with new equipment need to be improved.

Hysterectomy

- This is a major operation with serious risks, but very high satisfaction rates. Although hysterectomy is associated with a longer operating time and recovery period, and higher rates of post-operative complications, it offers permanent relief from heavy menstrual bleeding.
- The use of GnRH analogues for 3–4 months prior to fibroid surgery reduce both uterine volume and fibroid size. They are beneficial in the correction of pre-operative iron deficiency anaemia, if present, and reduce intra-operative blood loss. If myomectomy is planned with a midline incision, this can be converted to a pfannenstiel incision in many women with the use of GnRH analogues. If fertility has to be preserved, hsyteroscopic resection of the fibroids may be performed to treat submucous fibroids. For patients undergoing hysterectomy, a vaginal procedure is more likely following the use of these agents.

⚠ **Abnormal bleeding**

Non-menstrual vaginal bleeding is a distressing symptom. It could be due to an organic cause such as an endometrial polyp, or dysfunctional when no obvious pathology is found. It has numerous causes which vary with the age group of the patient.

One could divide these patients into 5 age groups; the first category till puberty (childhood); from puberty to 20 years (adolescent); 20–45 years (reproductive age group); 45–52 years (perimenopausal age group); and the postmenopausal age group.

Childhood

Any bleeding in this age group is likely to be of traumatic origin. This could be either due to an accident or unfortunately a result of child abuse. These children are normally very scared and should be looked after very sensitively. It is important to gain confidence by building a good rapport. This begins by consulting the child along with the parents in a very child-friendly atmosphere. It is best to avoid too many doctors visiting the child; hence an appropriately trained senior clinician should attend. Colourful rooms, toys, and sweets could be a helpful start. A history should be obtained from the parents. They may not have been present at the time of the episode, but it is important to know if they have accepted the explanation offered by the school or nursery etc. where the accident may have happened. It helps to know if anybody has witnessed the accident. If the circumstances leading to the symptom are suspicious, then the legal implications must be considered very carefully. It is essential to have a multidisciplinary approach. The paediatric team is likely to involve the appropriate social bodies to investigate the matter further.

The most likely accidental cause for these injuries is cycling, swimming, or playing in the garden.

After obtaining a detailed history, one must examine the child. This can be very difficult and should be done with the help of additional staff who can try to distract the child and at the same time be present as a witness. In most cases these injuries are superficial lacerations that cause spotting. These can be assessed by inspection. If the extent of the injury cannot be assessed or is deep, then the child may have to be assessed under anaesthesia. One may have to use a fine hysteroscope to visualize the inner vaginal area.

In most cases the lacerations tend to heal without any further active treatment. If the cut is deep, then it should be sutured under an anaesthetic.

Adolescent

Any abnormal bleeding in this age group is almost always dysfunctional. It is mainly due to hypothalamic dysfunction, or delayed, or failed ovulation. The bleeding could be irregular and occasionally heavy. A detailed history of the presenting symptoms and other relevant medical conditions is obtained. This is then followed by a thorough general and pelvic examination. It is not mandatory to perform a pelvic examination as the patient may not be sexually active and can be very embarrassing for the young patient. The prognosis is good as nearly 50% would resolve spontaneously in 2 years, and about 75% in 10 years. In patients with severe and persistent bleeding, it is important to rule out systemic causes such as bleeding disorders and hypothyroidism. If the clinical suspicion of an organic cause is high, then investigations such as blood tests and ultrasound examination must be considered. In almost all cases the treatment is conservative with the help of medications. Combined oral contraceptive pill is the first choice in most patients. Apart from regularizing the cycles and controlling the blood loss, the contraceptive effect is also helpful in this age group. Progesterone therapy during the luteal phase from day 15–25 of the cycle can be tried. These hormonal options could be tried in a cyclical manner for 4–6 months. In presence of heavy bleeding, tranexamic acid could be given on the days when bleeding is heaviest. In presence of painful periods, mefenamic acid could be beneficial. There is no need to investigate these patients routinely as the majority would resolve spontaneously and carcinoma is very unlikely in this age group.

Reproductive age group
Causes
- Abnormal bleeding between 20–40 years age is most likely due to benign disease such as endocervical or endometrial polyp, pelvic inflammatory disease, or a pregnancy complication such as an ectopic pregnancy or a miscarriage.
- Physiological causes include cervical ectropion or a mid-cycle ovulatory bleed.
- Dysfunctional uterine bleeding (DUB) is also common and the diagnosis is made by ruling out an organic cause.
- Hormonal therapy such as oral contraceptive pill could lead to irregular bleeding initially.
- Vaginal tears during intercourse and rape are the traumatic causes of abnormal bleeding.
- Vaginal, cervical, and endometrial cancers are very unlikely, but these should always be suspected.

Diagnosis
History
- A detailed history of the presenting and the associated symptoms is essential. Most patients in this age group present with either intermenstrual bleeding or post-coital bleeding. Associated symptoms such as vaginal discharge and pelvic pain could indicate pelvic infection. Weight loss, haematuria, and rectal bleeding could be indicators of invasive malignant disease.
- Regular cyclical bleeding suggests ovulatory DUB. It is commonly caused by benign organic disease such as fibromyomas and is considered favorable. Irregular acyclical bleeding is characteristic of organic disease, particularly cervical or endometrial carcinoma.
- A detailed gynaecological history should look for past gynaecological problems including abnormal smears, contraceptive history, and the fertility status.

- Obstetric history helps to know of any current or recent pregnancy. Cervical ectropion is seen in pregnancy. If there is a high suspicion of ectopic pregnancy risk factors must be noted.
- History relating to smoking, social status, and multiple sexual partners is helpful to assess the risk of cervical cancer.

Clinical examination
- General examination:
  - tired, exhausted looks, and anaemia reflect the severity of the blood loss.
  - cachexia, anaemia, and enlarged lymph nodes could be suggestive of underlying carcinoma.
- Pelvic examination:
  - vulval, vaginal, and cervical inspection should be performed to look for any obvious local lesions responsible for the bleeding.
  - cervical polyps, growths, ectropion, or purulent discharge may be seen on speculum examination.
  - bimanual examination helps to detect tenderness suggestive of ectopic pregnancy or pelvic infection. Hard, non-mobile mass is suggestive of carcinoma with a possibility of spread.

Investigations
- FBC may reflect the severity of the blood loss.
- If infection is suspected, it is very helpful to obtain high vaginal and endocervical swabs.
- A smear should be obtained if one is due. In the presence of obvious cervical lesions, a biopsy is helpful to establish a tissue diagnosis.
- Transvaginal ultrasound examination may be indicated to rule out ectopic pregnancy and to look for other organic pathologies such as endometrial or endocervical polyps. A pregnancy test is essential.
- Endometrial sampling is essential after the age of 40 years to look for any endometrial abnormality.
- Hysteroscopic examination may be required on the basis of the clinical findings or the ultrasound examination.

Treatment
- This would depend on the underlying cause.
- General measures include maintaining a menstrual calendar and iron therapy.
- Dysfunctional uterine bleeding could be treated using hormonal preparations such as the combined pill or progesterone. Prostaglandin synthetase inhibitors such as mefenamic acid or antifibrinolytics such as tranexamic acid are useful to treat ovulatory DUB.
- If ectopic pregnancy is detected, then medical or surgical treatment could be instituted. Surgical treatment could be laparoscopic or open, salpingotomy or salpingectomy.
- If pelvic infection is diagnosed, then appropriate antibiotic treatment is initiated.
- Symptomatic ectropion could be treated in the clinic using cryocautery, if the smears are normal.

- Symptomatic endocervical or endometrial polyps or fibroids may have to be removed surgically. A small cervical polyp could be avulsed in the clinic, but if in doubt about the origin or its vascularity, the polypectomy should be done under an anaesthetic. Further treatment in these patients is guided by the histology report.
- If a malignancy is diagnosed, then the treatment should be undertaken by the gynaecological oncologist in a multi-disciplinary manner.

Perimenopausal bleeding

After the age of 45 years any abnormal bleeding must be taken very seriously and investigated fully. It is most commonly anovulatory dysfunctional bleeding, but organic cause such as fibromyoma could be responsible. Cervical and endometrial carcinomas are more likely and these should be excluded.

The principles of investigation and treatment are the same as in postmenopausal bleeding. Transvaginal ultrasound examination, hysteroscopy, and endometrial sampling should be used to rule out sinister causes.

Postmenopausal bleeding

This is defined as any bleeding per vaginum 6 months or more after the cessation of menstrual periods. Most women with this symptom do not have any serious underlying abnormality, but it is the presenting symptom of an endometrial carcinoma.

Causes

- Malignant causes include vulval, vaginal, cervical, or endometrial cancers. Uterine sarcomas, fallopian tube cancer and oestrogen secreting tumour of the ovary are other rare cancers.
- Benign endometrial and endocervical polyps are very common in this age group.
- Atrophic vaginitis and urethral caruncle are due to oestrogen deficiency states.
- Vaginal or endometrial infections.
- Hormone replacement therapy, tamoxifen, and IUCD are iatrogenic causes.
- Trauma from intercourse and ring pessary lead to bleeding due to atrophy.

Diagnosis

History

- A detailed history of the presenting symptom and the associated symptoms is essential. Postmenopausal bleeding could be associated with vaginal discharge. Abdominal mass and weight loss are indicative of advanced malignant disease.
- History of any past gynaecological diseases, smear history, and contraceptive history is helpful.
- Obstetric history—incidence of endometrial carcinoma is higher in nulliparous women.
- Medical history particularly to look for diabetes, hypertension, or morbid obesity is important. Women with endometrial cancer are more likely to have these conditions and also they have surgical implications in terms of fitness.

- Prolonged unopposed oestrogen therapy is associated with increased risk of endometrial cancer. It is also important to note any history of taking hormone replacement therapy which could be the cause of bleeding in this age.

Clinical examination
- A thorough general examination is performed to look for cachexia and lymph node enlargement which suggest cancer.
- This is followed by abdominal and pelvic examination. Large uterine fibroids or advanced stage of endometrial cancer could present with a palpable mass in the abdomen.
- Speculum examination is performed to look for any local cause such as vaginitis, polyps, or other cervical abnormality.
- Bimanual examination helps in determining the uterine size, mobility, and tenderness. The uterus could be enlarged due to fibroids or advanced endometrial cancer. Lack of mobility suggests the spread of cancer, and tenderness is indicative of pelvic infection.

Investigations
- FBC is performed to look for anaemia. Raised white cell count is seen in infections and malignant disease.
- High vaginal and endocervical swabs are obtained if infection is suspected.
- Cervical smear must be done if one is due
- Transvaginal ultrasound is then performed to detect any obvious intrauterine pathology and to determine the endometrial thickness. If the endometrium is <5 mm thick, it is reassuring.
- If the thickness is >5 mm, then an endometrial sample should be sent for histology.
- If an intrauterine pathology is seen, then saline infusion sonography or hysteroscopy should be performed. An endometrial sample must be obtained.
- It is now possible to perform all of the above investigations in the outpatient settings that simplify the management of these patients. One-stop clinics are very popular in modern gynaecological practice.

Treatment
- This depends on the underlying cause.
- If endometrial histology is normal, hysteroscopic polypectomy of an endometrial polyp could be sufficient.
- Local oestrogen cream application could treat atrophic vaginitis.
- If endometrial cancer is diagnosed then this must be treated by the gynaecological oncologist with the help of radiotherapist and the specialist team.
- Early detection may allow surgical treatment. For advanced cases, radiotherapy may be the treatment of choice. Total abdominal hysterectomy with bilateral salpingo-oophorectomy ± pelvic and aortic lymphadenectomy is the traditional surgical treatment for endometrial cancer.

Hints

- Vaginal bleeding in children is almost always traumatic.
- One must rule out the possibility of child abuse.
- Non-menstrual vaginal bleeding in the adolescent age group is likely to be of dysfunctional nature.
- Intermenstrual or post-coital bleeding in the reproductive age group is likely to be due to a benign underlying cause.
- Conservative treatment may be adequate for regular bleeding and could include medical treatment, Mirena coil, or endometrial ablative surgery.
- Patients with peri- and postmenopausal bleeding can now be investigated in the outpatient settings using endometrial samplers, transvaginal ultrasound, and outpatient hysteroscopy.
- After 40 years of age, any abnormal bleeding must be thoroughly investigated due to the possibility of an underlying carcinoma.
- Conservative treatment is commonly used for benign pathology, but the chances of hysterectomy are higher in those who do not respond adequately.

⑦ Menstrual cramps

A painful period ± nausea and vomiting is a common symptom in the reproductive age group. This can occur without an underlying organic pathology (primary dysmenorrhoea) or with an underlying pathology (secondary dysmenorrhoea).

Causes

- *Primary dysmenorrhoea*: this occurs at menarche and is likely to be associated with ovulatory cycles. There is no detectable organic cause in these patients.
- *Secondary dysmenorrhoea*: this is associated with an underlying cause such as fibroid, adenomyosis, endometriosis, pelvic infections and IUCD. This occurs at a later stage in the reproductive life.

Diagnosis

History

- The age of the patient helps in knowing the possible cause for the painful periods.
- Pain during the 1st and 2nd day of the period at menarche is likely to suggest primary dysmenorrhoea.
- Premenstrual pain, or pain throughout the period, suggests an underlying organic cause.
- A particular note about the use of analgesia and any form of hormonal treatment should be made.
- Associated symptoms such as menorrhagia, irregular cycles, dyspareunia, and vaginal discharge should be noted.
- Other than the detailed menstrual history and the associated symptoms, it is important to note the current contraceptive needs, the smear history and the details of any past pregnancies.
- A stenosed cervix could lead to secondary dysmenorrhoea.
- It is also important to obtain a complete medical and surgical history.

Primary dysmenorrhoea

It could be ovulatory or anovulatory and is mainly caused by uterine muscle spasm or by prostaglandin release.

- Ovulatory cycles are regular and may also have pain in the middle of the cycle (mittelschmerz).
- Anovulatory cycles are common during the initial months after menarche and in the perimenopausal age group. The periods are likely to be irregular and heavy.

Secondary dysmenorrhoea

This is likely to have other associated symptoms.

- The pain with endometriosis is likely to start premenstrually and could persist during the period.
- Deep dyspareunia could suggest endometriosis, pelvic infections or fibroids.
- Offensive vaginal discharge could be present in patients with pelvic inflammatory disease.
- IUCD could cause crampy pain by itself or by causing a pelvic infection.

Examination

- *General examination*: one must look for any obvious signs of distress or pallor.
- *Abdominal examination*: guarding, rebound tenderness, and tenderness. The location of tenderness and palpable masses should be noted.
- *Speculum examination*: to look for IUCD, vaginal discharge and if present, obtain swabs.
- *Bimanual examination*: this is performed to look for uterine size, tenderness and mobility. Nodules in the uterosacral ligaments and any palpable fibroids should be noted. Uterine immobility could be suggestive of endometriosis or pelvic inflammatory disease.

Investigations

- FBC—to look for any raised white cell count or anaemia.
- C-reactive protein to look for any acute infections.
- Hormonal profile including serum FSH, LH, and testosterone may be useful if clinically indicated. Polycystic ovarian disease may be responsible for anovulatory dysmenorrhoea.
- Transvaginal ultrasound examination to look for any obvious pelvic pathology such as fibroids, ovarian cysts, or misplaced IUCD.
- Laparoscopy and hysteroscopy should be considered if symptoms continue or the ultrasound scan suggests a pelvic pathology.

Treatment

Primary dysmenorrhoea

- NSAIDs—mefenamic acid 500 mg 8 hrly, 24–48 hr prior to the onset of the pain and to be continued during the most painful days of the period. NSAIDs are an effective treatment for dysmenorrhoea, though women using them need to be aware of the significant risk of adverse effects. Ibuprofen 400 mg 8 hrly is commonly used. Paracetamol may be tried in some cases of mild dysmenorrhoea. The above analgesics tend to help women with anovulatory dysmenorrhoea.
- Combined oral contraceptive pill—this is useful to treat women with ovulatory dysmenorrhoea. It may have to be combined with NSAIDs to achieve better pain control. These medications could be tried for about 12 months. 80% of women with primary dysmenorrhoea are likely to respond favourably. If no relief is seen, then further investigations should be undertaken. A laparoscopy in these circumstances is likely to detect an underlying abnormality such as endometriosis or pelvic infection.
- When medical treatment fails, surgery has been an option. Uterine nerve ablation (UNA) and presacral neurectomy (PSN) are 2 surgical treatments that have become increasingly utilised in recent years. Both procedures interrupt the majority of the cervical sensory nerve fibres, thus diminishing uterine pain. However both operations only partially interrupt some of the cervical sensory nerve fibres in the pelvic area; therefore dysmenorrhoea associated with additional pelvic pathology may not always benefit from this type of surgery. There is insufficient evidence to recommend the use of nerve interruption in the management of dysmenorrhoea, regardless of cause.

Secondary dysmenorrhoea
- The treatment would depend on the underlying cause. This may include medical or surgical management of endometriosis if found.
- Treatment with antibiotics if pelvic infection is detected.
- Medical or surgical management of fibroids may be necessary.
- If an IUCD is present, the pain could be treated with NSAIDs. In case of infection, the IUCD may have to be removed and patient treated with broad spectrum antibiotics.

Hints
- Dysmenorrhoea is a common debilitating symptom faced by many women in the reproductive age group.
- In 50% the symptoms are moderate and in a further 10–15% it can be severe.
- Majority of women (over 80%) with primary dysmenorrhoea benefit from NSAIDs.
- Combined pill is a good second line treatment.
- Treatment of secondary dysmenorrhoea depends on the underlying pathology.

Chronic and acute abdominal pain

Sandeep Mane

Barry Whitlow

⑦ Chronic abdominal pain

It is one of the common presenting complaints accounting for about 10% of referrals to the gynaecology outpatient clinic. Majority of the times no obvious pathology is detected. It is important to manage these patients with sensitivity to ensure that the resulting psychological damage is limited. At the same time the clinician should avoid getting forced into undertaking investigations that are not clinically indicated.

Causes

Gynaecological

● *Pelvic infection*

Recurrent infections with resulting adhesion formation could become a difficult clinical problem to treat.

● *Endometriosis*

Is one of the commonest reasons for ongoing pelvic pain. It affects approximately 10% of women in reproductive age. Unfortunately, the pathophysiology is still poorly understood and it is not easy to clinically correlate the presenting symptoms with the severity of the disease as seen at laparoscopy. There is a range of symptoms and most commonly women present with pelvic pain, dysmenorrhoea, infertility, or a pelvic mass. Direct visualization and biopsy during laparoscopy or laparotomy is the gold standard diagnostic test for this condition and enables the gynaecologist to identify the location, extent, and severity of the disease.

● *Tumour*

Pelvic tumours, benign and malignant, could lead to long-standing unresolved pain. Ovarian cysts and fibroids are the commonest tumours responsible for such pain.

● *Other causes*

Ovulatory pain (mittelschmerz) and premenstrual pain are the physiological causes for chronic pain. Pelvic congestion syndrome is being accepted as another possible cause.

Non gynaecological

● *Depression*

This could be a cause for chronic pain and also an effect of long-standing pain for which no cause can be found. It is a diagnosis by exclusion.

● *Childhood sexual abuse*

Childhood trauma can present with chronic pain.

● *Urinary tract infection*

Recurrent UTIs could lead to chronic cystitis and unresolving pain.

● *Irritable bowel disease*

This is a very common cause and is diagnosed by exclusion.

● *Inflammatory bowel disease*

Crohn's disease or ulcerative colitis can both lead to chronic pain.

● *Constipation*

This is not uncommon and can be treated effectively if detected.

Symptoms

Pelvic pain

A detailed history about the onset duration and progress of the pain is essential. This will provide significant information to help arrive at the diagnosis.

Associated symptoms

These include dyspareunia, vaginal discharge, bladder, and bowel symptoms. Dyspareunia could be caused by endometriosis or pelvic infection. Offensive vaginal discharge is suggestive of pelvic infection.

Other relevant history

- Detailed menstrual history, contraceptive history, and smear history is essential.
- History about any previous pregnancies. Any traumatic deliveries and postnatal depression could be the underlying reason for chronic pelvic pain.
- Previous medical and surgical history to note any bowel and bladder related problems in the past.
- History of medications such as analgesics used in the past provides information about the severity of pain.
- Social history—unemployment and drug abuse could be important social problems leading to depression and symptoms such as chronic pelvic pain.
- Effect of the symptoms on the patient's lifestyle—absence from work and disturbance in family life may reflect the severity of pain.

Signs

- *General examination*

While obtaining history and performing general examination it is important to observe the patient for expressions of being in obvious pain and discomfort.

- *Abdominal examination*

This is done to look for previous scars indicating multiple surgeries to remove vestigial organs. Loaded sigmoid may suggest constipation. Any tender areas in the abdomen may suggest intra-abdominal pathology.

- *Pelvic examination*
- *Vulval inspection*

This is performed to look for any obvious discharge.

- *Speculum examination*

This would reveal any offensive vaginal discharge suggesting pelvic infection or presence of local lesions on the cervix or the vagina.

- *Bimanual examination*

To look for forniceal thickening and tenderness. Nodules and tenderness in the uterosacral ligaments may indicate endometriosis. Any obvious palpable masses may be due to tumours or fibroids. Rectal examination may reveal a loaded rectum suggesting constipation.

Investigations
• *Full blood count*
It is important to look for raised white cell count suggesting presence of infection.
• *Raised C-reactive protein*
This is seen in the presence of pelvic infections and inflammatory bowel disease.
• *Urine culture and sensitivity*
To look for evidence of urinary tract infection.
• *Endocrine profile*
This could help to detect raised LH/FSH ratio and serum testosterone levels suggesting polycystic ovarian disease.
• *Transvaginal ultrasound examination*
It is very useful to detect any obvious pelvic pathology such as uterine fibroid, ovarian cyst, endometriotic cyst, and polycystic ovaries. A normal scan is also very reassuring and leads to symptom relief in the anxious patients.
• *Diagnostic laparoscopy*
Depending on the severity of the symptoms and the findings of the preliminary investigations one may have to perform a laparoscopy to evaluate the abdomen and pelvis further. It is an invasive test associated with anaesthetic and surgical risks, but provides valuable information to understand the cause of the chronic pain. A negative laparoscopy also becomes very reassuring and can help the anxious patient psychologically.

Treatment
Non-gynaecological cause
• A systematic approach and extreme sensitivity is necessary throughout the management of these patients.
• One must think of non-gynaecological causes, which are likely to cause chronic pelvic pain.
• Psychological disturbances are common and counselling could benefit these patients significantly.
• Dietary alterations to increase the dietary fibre content along with increased daily fluid intake should be considered.
• Stool softeners and other laxatives such as Senokot Hi-Fibre can cure pelvic pain caused by constipation.
• If clinically indicated, referral should be considered for the opinion of a bowel surgeon at an early stage.

Gynaecological cause
• If a gynaecological cause is found, then appropriate medical or surgical treatment is initiated.
• If regular analgesics do not work and the routine investigations have failed to detect a specific cause, a referral to the pain clinic should be considered.
• Laparoscopy should be considered only if necessary. Surgical therapy can be performed concurrently with diagnostic surgery and may include excision or ablation of endometriotic tissue, division of adhesions, and removal of endometriotic cysts. Laparoscopic excision

or ablation of endometriosis has been shown to be effective in the management of pain in mild-to-moderate endometriosis. Adjunctive medical treatment pre- or postoperatively may prolong the symptom-free interval. There is insufficient evidence from the studies identified to conclude that hormonal suppression in association with surgery for endometriosis is associated with a significant benefit with regard to any of the outcomes identified. There is little or no difference in the effectiveness of GnRHas in comparison with other medical treatments for endometriosis. Side effects of GnRHas can be controlled by the addition of addback therapy.

Hints

- It is a common problem and can be difficult to solve.
- Patients need to be treated with utmost sensitivity.
- Underlying psychological factor must be explored.
- Multidisciplinary approach may be more effective.

Acute abdominal pain

Definition
Pain that is rapid in onset (<24 hr) usually associated with signs of peritonism (guarding, rebound, rigidity).

Gynaecological causes[1]
- Common: ectopic pregnancy, miscarriage, ovarian cyst, pelvic inflammatory disease.
- Less common: Ovarian/adnexal torsion/tubovarian abscess.

History
LMP, site of pain and nature ?colicky or persistent ?vaginal discharge ?fever ?previous past gynaecology history.

Examination
Abdomen soft or rigid, ?rebound, ?peritonism when coughs, ?requiring regular analgesia, ?mass palpated.

Investigations
Pregnancy test, MSU for microscopy and culture, high vaginal swab for culture (HVS), endocervical swabs, FBC, serum human chorionic gonad-otrophin (HCG), G&S, pelvic ultrasound (US) examination.

Diagnosis
- *Ectopic:* serum HCG >1500 U empty uterus on ultrasound with small amount of per vaginal bleeding and adnexal pain. Transvaginal scan (TVS) can diagnose 80% cases and laparoscopy almost 100% cases.
- *Miscarriage:* colicky pelvic pain with per vaginal bleeding moderate/large amount, positive pregnancy test and US suggests miscarriage.
- *Ovarian cyst:* usually constant pain and cyst is seen on US. May be a simple cyst, or have mixed echos of haemorrhage (spider web appearance)—haemorrhagic cysts classically luteal phase cycle and after intercourse. Ground glass appearance on US suggests endometrioma and mixed bright echos suggest a dermoid.
- *Ovarian cyst/fibroid torsion:* pain constant or colicky may radiate to leg, associated with vomiting and raised white cell count (WCC) or inter-leukin 6 (IL6[2]), cyst seen on US. Doppler ultrasound maybe useful.
- *Pelvic inflammatory disease (PID):* acute PID associated with pyrexia (>38°C), cervical excitation/dyspareunia, vaginal discharge, and raised WCC/C-reactive proteins (CRP). Gold standard diagnosis is at laparo-scopy, but usually not required and is first treated medically. If non responsive to IV treatment consider tubovarian abscess and drainage.
- *Non-gynaecological causes* should be considered and computerized tomography (CT) is a useful tool[3].

Treatment
- *Ectopic:* laparoscopic salpingectomy if contralateral tube healthy and patient is haemodynamically stable. Conservative approaches can be considered in specific situations.

- *Miscarriage:* evacuation of retained products of conception (ERPC) or conservative management. Medical management can be offered provided patient is haemodynamically stable.
- *Ovarian cyst:* when <5 cm and not requiring regular analgesia, it can be managed conservatively. If patient requires parenteral analgesia and/or there are signs of acute abdomen then laparoscopy and ovarian cystectomy may be advisable.
- *Haemorrhagic ovarian cysts:* haemorrhage into a cyst is usually managed conservatively provided it is not causing a lot of pain and the patient is haemodynamically stable. If pain is not controlled, signs of peritonism or haemodynamic disturbance, laparoscopic lavage is performed and a cystectomy or haemostatic manoeuvre employed[4].
- *Ovarian cyst torsion:* torsion can be managed conservatively by laparoscopically untwisting the torsion if employed within 36 hr of the torsion, thus avoiding adnexectomy[5].
- *PID:* oral treatment: ofloxacin 400 mg twice a day plus oral metronidazole 400 mg twice a day for 14 days. IV treatment: ofloxacin 400 mg bd plus metronidazole 500 mg tds for 14 days. Oral therapy can be started 24 hr after clinical improvement. Surgical drainage may be rarely required.

References

1. Burnett LS (1988). Gynecologic causes of the acute abdomen. *Surgical Clinics of North America*, **68**(2), 385–98.
2. Cohen SB, Wattiez A, Stockheim D, *et al.* (2001). The accuracy of serum interleukin-6 and tumour necrosis factor as markers for ovarian torsion. *Human Reproduction*, **16**(10), 2195–7.
3. Taourel P, Pradel J, Fabre JM. *et al.* (1995). Role of CT in the acute nontraumatic abdomen. *Seminars in Ultrasound, CT & MR*, **16**(2), 151–64.
4. Larue L, Barau C, Rigonnot L. *et al.* (1991).Rupture of hemorrhagic ovarian cysts. Value of celioscopic surgery. *Journal de Gynecologie, Obstetrique et Biologie de la Reproduction*, **20**(7), 928–32.
5. Rody A, Jackisch C, Klockenbusch W. *et al.* (2002). The conservative management of adnexal torsion—a case-report and review of the literature. *European Journal of Obstetrics, Gynecology, & Reproductive Biology*, **101**(1), 83–6.

Intra-operative emergencies

Barry Whitlow

☠ Haemorrhage

A blood loss of >500 ml at any gynaecological operation is considered significant by the RCOG clinical governance standards. When estimated blood loss has occurred intra-operatively the following measures may be considered:

Treatment

1. Inform your anaesthetist and ask for cross-match of 4–6 units of blood.
2. Careful ligation of appropriate vessels with sutures.
3. Careful use of diathermy and consider using Surgicel™.
4. To apply pressure with a warm pack and ensure adequate blood and or clotting factors with the on call haematologist and send a clotting screen.
5. Rarely the organ bleeding (tube, ovary, or uterus) will require removing surgically to arrest bleeding.
6. Very rarely consider ligation (but not division) of anterior division of internal iliac possibly with vascular surgeon on call.[1] A vascular clamp/or bulldog clamp can be used to see if ligation of the iliac artery will be useful or not.
7. Should there be one available, an interventional radiologist can be called to locate and occlude the vessels causing the haemorrhage when other measures have failed. Cell savers when used may reduce available clotting factors.[2]
8. The use of the protease inhibitor aprotinin, arginine vasopressin derivatives (DDAVP), and recombinant factor VII (rfVIIa) can all be considered when blood loss continues despite the above measures and have been proven to be useful.[3]
9. Very rarely a pack may be left in situ and removed at second look laparotomy 24 hours later, especially when hypothermia (<35 degrees C), acidosis > 7.2, coagulopathy PTT > 16 sec exists.[4]

References

1. Oleszczuk D, Cebulak K, Skret A, et al. (1995). Long term observation of patients after bilateral ligation of internal iliac arteries. *Ginekologia Polska*, **66**(9), 533–6.
2. Guo XY, Duan H, Wang JJ, et al. (2004). Effect of intraoperative using cell saver on blood sparing and its impact on coagulation function. *Acta academiae medicinae sinicae* **26**(2); 188–91, 2004.
3. Paramo JA, Lecumberri R, Hernandez M, et al. (2004). Pharmacological alternatives to blood transfusion: what is new about? *Medicina Clinica*, **122**(6), 231–6.
4. Stagnitti F, Bresadola L, Calderale SM (2003). Abdominal "packing": indications and method. *Annali Italiani di Chirurgia*, **74**(5), 535–42.

☠ Perforated uterus

This may occur during D&C, hysteroscopy, insertion of a coil, or at ERPC/suction termination of pregnancy (STOP). It may be noticed at the time by the feeling of 'lack of resistance' when probing the uterine cavity or may present postoperatively with signs of acute abdomen. Its incidence is 0.1–0.5% and risk of associated bowel trauma is > 0.1%[1].

Treatment

1. Inform your anaesthetist and ensure a large-bore cannula is inserted.
2. Leave instrument in the uterus that you believe has caused perforation and, if this is a suction cannula, then turn off the suction.
3. Proceed to a laparoscopy, assuming the patient is haemodynamically stable.
4. Inspect uterus for perforations/bleeding points and if possible inspect as much intestine at the laparoscopy as you can. If in doubt about bowel trauma, especially if fat which may be part of the omentum was sucked or removed, patient needs a laparotomy for a good evaluation. Call a colorectal surgeon.
5. Commonly small perforations that are not bleeding and can be managed conservatively with antibiotics (cefuroxime and metronidazole) and admitted overnight for observation.
6. Should there be bleeding from the uterus then a laparoscopic suture or laparotomy may be needed to repair the perforation and to arrest bleeding[2–4].
7. ERPC or STOP can then be completed under laparoscopic control and under ultrasound guidance to ensure no retained POCs[5].

References

1. Lindell G, Flam F (1995). Management of uterine perforations in connection with legal abortions. *Acta Obstetricia et Gynecologica Scandinavica*, **74**(5), 373–5.
2. Sharma JB, Malhotra M, Pundir P (2003). Laparoscopic oxidized cellulose (Surgicel) application for small uterine perforations. *International Journal of Gynaecology & Obstetrics*, **83**(3), 271–5.
3. Mustafa MS, Gurab S (1995). Endoscopic management of bleeding uterine perforation occurring during evacuation of retained products of conception. *International Journal of Gynaecology & Obstetrics*, **49**(1), 71–2.
4. Romer T, Lober R (1998). Endoscopic management of uterine perforation with the ENDO-UNIVERSAL surgical stapler. *Zentralblatt fur Gynakologie*, **120**(2), 69–70.
5. Kohlenberg CF, Casper GR (1996). The use of intraoperative ultrasound in the management of a perforated uterus with retained products of conception. *Australian & New Zealand Journal of Obstetrics & Gynaecology*, **36**(4), 482–4.

☠ Damage to urinary tract/blood vessels/bowel

Urinary tract trauma

Damage to the urinary tract should ideally be recognized at the time of surgery. Postoperative vaginal leakage of urine, urine in drainage bottles, or the presence of loin pain should always raise the possibility of inadvertent damage to the urinary tract.

If there is trauma to the ureter or base of the bladder during surgery, the on call consultant urologist should be called to theatre. For trauma to the bladder dome a two layer closure using 2/0 Vicryl should be performed followed by methylene blue dye to check for leakage.

If the ureter is damaged and noted during surgery then, depending on the site of damage to the ureter, the following maybe considered: ureteric reimplantation, Boari flap, or ileal conduit. These procedures should be carried out by a consultant urologist.

Should the urinary tract trauma be diagnosed in the postoperative period, then:

- *For suspected bladder trauma:* a speculum examination may reveal the point of leakage. If not identifiable, a catheter is inserted and methylene blue dye instilled and a swab test performed. Non-colouration, but soaking of the swab will indicate ureteric fistula and swabs soaked with blue indicate vesicovaginal fistula. Alternatively a cystogram with radio-opaque material can be performed which will reveal the point of leakage.
- *For suspected ureteric trauma:* an intravenous urogram can be performed and hydronephrosis and delayed emptying or even complete renal obstruction can be seen. Usually in such cases loin pain is evident within 6–12 hours after surgery and a percutaneous nephrostomy should be performed as a primary procedure to avoid damage to that kidney. Urea and electrolytes may not be abnormal if the damage is only on one side.

Trauma to blood vessels

These mostly occur during laparoscopic procedures.

Trauma to large vessels (aorta, vena cava, iliac vein/artery)

This is usually during laparoscopy by either the verres needle or the trocar. Should trauma be suspected (blood returning up needle/trocar) the following management should ensue:

- Leave the trocar/needle in situ and ensure no gas is running in.
- Place patient in steep Trendelenberg position.
- Cross-match 6 U and ask for 2 U of O negative blood/maintain adequate fluid replacement.
- Perform a midline laparotomy and apply considerable pressure proximal to the vessel injury to slow down blood loss.
- Call for vascular surgeon to attend immediately to the emergency.

Trauma to pelvic side wall vessels/venous oozing

This can be encountered when performing laparoscopy and dividing adhesions.

- Indiscriminate use of diathermy should be avoided as this can lead to further bleeding and retroperitoneal haemorrhage.
- Pressure with a sucker or tonsil swab should be maintained for at least 2–3 min and careful lavage performed to ensure haemostasis.
- A redivac drain should be left in situ postoperatively.

Inferior epigastric injury

This should be avoided by careful inspection of the course of the epigastric vessels when inserting laparoscopic ports, but should the epigastric vessel be damaged then the following can be instituted;

- Pass a Foley catheter down the port site and inflate the balloon and pull back to apply pressure.
- Diathermy to the bleeding point via a contralateral port.
- Pass a suture around the vessel using a Grice or Bonney–Reverdin needle.
- Enlarge the port skin site and place a Vicryl suture directly through the sheath under laparoscopic vision.

Trauma to bowel

If perforation occurred with the *Verres needle* one may notice faeculent fluid during Palmers test or high inflation pressures and gas escaping from patient's anus.

- Verres needle should be left in situ.
- A laparotomy or alternatively another site for entry (e.g. Palmer's point entry using a 5 mm laparoscope could be performed to confirm the diagnosis).
- Should the diagnosis be confirmed then a general surgeon should be called for assistance.
- A suture should be placed laparoscopically or via laparotomy. If it involved large bowel then copius peritoneal lavage should be performed.
- Broad spectrum antibiotics should be given and the patient admitted for observation.

If noticed from the *trocar insertion* may notice faeculent smell or faeculent fluid via side port.

- Again trocar should be left in situ.
- A laparotomy or alternatively another site for entry (e.g. Palmer's point entry using a 5 mm laparoscope could be performed to confirm the diagnosis).
- Should laparotomy be performed then the umbilical port site can be extended along the length of the port to guide to the area of perforation. Should the diagnosis be confirmed then a general surgeon should be called for assistance.
- A suture placed laparoscopically or via laparotomy should be considered. If it involves large bowel copius peritoneal lavage should be performed.
- Broad spectrum antibiotics should be given and the patient admitted for observation.
- Consideration of defunctioning of the bowel should be considered, although is rarely required.

Postoperative complications

Barry Whitlow

Michelle Fynes

:☹: Postoperative collapse

Postoperative collapse is rare but requires very prompt action to avoid multisystem organ failure. The common causes/signs are:

- **Anoxia:** e.g. inhalation of vomit/obstruction of airway/pneumonia. Usually there will be central cyanosis and a dramatic drop in oxygen saturation with an obstruction visible in the airway.
- **Central circulatory failure:** myocardial infarction/pulmonary embolism. There may be preceding crushing/severe chest pain, raised JVP, or pulmonary oedema.
- **Sepsis:** hypotension and warm peripheries.
- **Drug causes:** overdose or anaphylactic reaction (opiates, antibiotics)— sudden or delayed reaction after giving medication.
- **Reactionary or secondary haemorrhage:** pulse rate will initially be raised with normal BP but then may fall abruptly if volume depletion is not corrected. Associated features of shock with cold peripheries will be noted followed by severe drop in BP. Loss of consciousness and cardiac arrhythmia indicates >30–40% of blood volume loss and severe shock.
- **Cerebral causes:** stroke, epilepsy—previous history or biting tongue/urinary incontinence and tonic/clonic sezures or focal hemiparesis/dysphasia.

Initial management

1. *Call for help*/pull emergency alarm.
2. *Assess airway*—clear/maintain patency. Apply 15 litres oxygen/min via tight-fitting face mask with reservoir bag and attach pulse oximeter. Ventilate with bag/mask/consider intubation if hypoxaemic.
3. *Assess circulation*/perform CPR if required and call crash team if needed. Attach ECG monitor/automated external defibrillator as per advance life support (ALS) protocol.
4. *Attach BP monitor.* Ensure good IV access and take bloods for FBC, UEs, glucose, cross-match, blood cultures, blood gases, and run intravenous infusion (IVI) with colloid initially.
5. Inform consultant in charge of case/call for senior help. Arrange chest X-ray.
6. Management thereafter will be dependent on cause.

☠ Postoperative chest pain

Causes/signs to aid diagnosis

- *Musculoskeletal pain*—often a specific point of tenderness that can be reproduced by touching the affected site with the examining finger.
- *Pleuritic chest pain*—pain on inspiration can be caused by musculoskeletal causes, pneumonia/pneumothorax or, more importantly, pulmonary embolus.
- *Central chest pain*—this can be caused by massive pulmonary embolus. When interscapular consider aortic dissection. Pain radiating from the chest to the jaw/arm obviously alerts one to the diagnosis of ischaemic heart disease.
- *Shoulder tip/apical chest pain*—common after a laparoscopy and occur after diagphragmatic irritation with CO_2 gas. This may be also related to haemoperitoneum.
- *Retrosternal chest pain* that settles after giving antacid indicates gastro-oesophageal reflux. Care should be exercised to exclude IHD and PE.

History

- Look at risk factors for causes e.g. risk of thromboembolic disease after operation >30min, obese, thrombophilia.
- Description of the pain (see above).

Examination

- Inspect—look for central cyanosis assess respiratory rate (abnormal > 20).
- Palpate for point tenderness and percuss for hyper-resonance of pneumothorax.
- Auscultate for reduced breath sounds in pneumothorax and signs of pulmonary oedema or pneumonia.

Investigations

- Oxygen saturation on air (normal >98%).
- Chest X-ray—pneumonia, pneumothorax, PE, rib fracture.
- Ventilation/perfusion (V:Q) scan or spiral CT/MRA for PE.
- FBC (raised WCC in pneumonia) + arterial blood gases (low oxygen saturation in PE), troponin measurement, consider D-dimers.
- ECG—tachycardia (and rarely S1 Q3 T3) in PE. ST changes with MI. Note pneumothorax can mimic signs of MI[1].

Treatment

- *Musculoskeletal pain*—physiotherapy and non-steroidal anti-inflammatory drugs (NSAIDs).
- *Pleuritic chest pain*—depends on cause:
  - pneumonia—antibiotics and NSAIDs
  - pneumothorax—conservative or aspiration/chest drain depending on degree of pneumothorax
  - pulmonary embolus—oxygen and heparin, rarely will further measures be required.

Central chest pain
interscapular and is aortic dissection consider lowering BP and refer to
cardiothoracic team.
- cardiac pain, angina—GTN, myocardial infarction—diamorphine
  2.5–5 mg IV with antiemetic.

Shoulder tip/apical chest pain—reassure and simple analgesia if
required.

Retrosternal chest pain—if diagnosis is gastro-oesophageal reflux, pre-
scribe Gaviscon™/magnesium trisilicate.

Reference

. Raev D (1996). A case of spontaneous left-sided pneumothorax with ECG changes resembling
acute myocardial infarction. *International Journal of Cardiology*, **56**(2), 197–9.

☼ Postoperative abdominal distension

Causes
- Haemorrhage
- Postoperative gastrointestinal ileus
- Acute gastric dilatation
- Intestinal obstruction
- Peritonitis
- Urinary retention
- Post-operative faecal impaction
- Gossypiboma.

Haemorrhage
- Usually following laparotomy or laparosocopy
- Check pulse and BP
- Appropriate resuscitation including IV access
- FBC, clotting, group and crossmatch
- Replacement blood products as appropriate
- Radiological or surgical intervention as appropriate to achieve haemostasis.

Postoperative ileus
- Common after a laparotomy
- Due to temporary depression of normal peristalsis of the gastrointestinal tract (GIT) secondary to manipulation
- GIT function normally returns 24–72 hr postoperatively
  - Gastric peristalsis: within 24–48 hr
  - Colonic activity: after 48 hr
- Symptoms: leads to mild abdominal distension and discomfort
- Examination: absent bowel sounds during first 48–72 hr
- Management: conservative!
  - nil by mouth
  - IV fluid replacement
  - nasogastric drainage if vomiting
- Return of normal peristaltic activity heralded by mild cramps, passage of flatus, and return of appetite
- If function does not return at this time, must consider a potentiating cause.

Acute gastric dilatation
- Usually follows overfilling of the stomach with fluid and gas.
- Common in malnourished, chronically immobilized patients, and asthmatics where oxygen masks were used in the immediate postoperative period.
- Fluid and air cause gross distension of the stomach.
- Onset is insidious.
- Symptoms:
  - may have severe pain and dyspnea and thus, mimic a myocardial infarction.
  - may be accompanied by sweating, hiccups, dehydration.

- Acid blood gases: hypochloremic metabolic alkalosis due to fluid and electrolyte loss into the stomach.
- Treatment: conservative
  - nasogastric tube to decompress
  - appropriate fluid replacement
  - monitor serum electrolytes and correct as appropriate.

Urinary retention

- Patient has poor urine output or unable to void.
- Patient may complain of suprapubic discomfort.
- If catheterized, check for blockage. May flush catheter or change indwelling catheter if necessary.
- If not catheterized, may perform intermittent catheterization or insert indwelling catheter depending on patient's status.
- Check for urinary tract infection and treat accordingly.

Postoperative fecal impaction

- Usually secondary to colonic ileus and impaired rectal sensation
- More common in the elderly
- Anticholinergic drugs and opiate analgesics may predispose
- Diagnosis: rectal examination
- Treatment: high-fiber diet, increased oral fluids, enemas, or manual removal under general anesthetic.

Intestinal obstruction

May be secondary to:
- Paralytic ileus
- Mechanical obstruction
- Peritonitis.

Paralytic Ileus common in patients with:
- Metabolic disturbances, e.g. hypokalemia
- Patients on tricyclic antidepressant
- Intraperitoneal inflammation
- Intraperitoneal hematomas.

Mechanical obstruction common in postoperative adhesions and internal hernia.

Peritonitis: may be secondary to:
- Bowel injury
  - may also occur after laparoscopy
  - *serious complication* if large perforation. May have high mortality rate.
  - may have small leak or develop into an abscess. Less dramatic signs and symptoms.
- Bladder injury
- Foreign body
- Infection (e.g. abscess).

Symptoms

- Similar to ileus. However, will experience an *initial unremarkable recovery* before obstruction manifests
- Pain
- Vomiting (points more to small bowel obstruction)
- Constipation/absolute
- Haematuria or blood per external meatus may point to bladder injury.

Examination

- Hyperactive, 'tinkling' bowel sounds
- If with peritonitis, may have severe systemic upset, generalized peritonism and guarding, absent bowel sounds.

Investigations

- Bloods: U&E, FBC, ABGs
- Plain films: air-fluid levels in loops of small bowel (erect X-ray centred to the diaphragm is valuable in making the diagnosis). If with bowel perforation, will show gas under diaphragm
- Small bowel follow through: if former is equivocal
- Ultrasound: can be used to differentiate paralytic ileus from mechanical obstruction as the peristaltic movement of the bowels in the latter is observed. May also visualize intra-abdominal foreign body, abscess, fluid in cul-de-sac (blood, pus, urine)
- Cystography or retrograde urethrography: if bladder injury is suspected
- CT/MRI: for deep abscess.

Management

- IV fluid resuscitation
- Decompression with a nasogastric tube
- Careful monitoring of BP, HR, respiration, temperature
- Hourly urinary monitoring
- Consider central venous line
- If with *small leak from bowel injury*, may consider radiologic guided placement of a large-bore drain into any collection. Periodic irrigation then performed.
- Above conservative measure are satisfactory if:
  - reduction of pain
  - nasogastric aspirate becomes cleaner and volumes reduce
  - reduced abdominal distension
  - passage of flatus
- Consider laparotomy or laparoscopy if:
  - conservative treatment ineffective after 48 hr.
  - remove foreign body
  - *large leaks from bowel injury or with signs of peritonism*
  - *TENDERNESS* is an indication for urgent or early surgery.
- If intra-abdominal abscess, start empiric antibiotics. May be drained guided by interventional radiology. If unresponsive, may require drainage via laparoscopy or laparotomy.

- If with bladder injury but
  - with *small leaks*: conservative treatment with indwelling catheter
  - with *large damage*: bladder repair with subsequent catheter placement

Gossypiboma

- Tumor-like presentation of an operative sponge left by accident during a laparotomy. Patient may be asymptomatic except for abdominal enlargement.
- Diagnosis: plain abdominal X-ray is unhelpful. Detected by ultrasonography or CT scan.
- Treatment: re-exploration and removal of foreign body. May also be laparoscopically removed.

ⓘ Postoperative pyrexia

Definition

The Center for Disease Control has defined postoperative pyrexia as a temperature of 100.4°F or 38°C or greater on any 2 postoperative days excluding the first 24 hours.

Causes

- Postoperative pyrexia is a common complication after a gynecologic procedure.
- It occurs in 25% of women after an abdominal hysterectomy and in 35% of women after a vaginal hysterectomy.
- The causes can be infectious or non-infectious in origin.
- The onset of fever can help determine the possible cause.

Within 24 hours	24 to 48 hours	3–5 days	5–7 days	7–10 days
• Metabolic response	• Respiratory (bacterial or aspiration pneumonia)	• Urinary tract infection	• Intra-abdominal abscess	• Wound infections
• Atelectasis				
• Necrotizing streptococcal & clostridial wound infection	• Catheter-related		• Deep venous thrombosis	
	• Persistent atelectasis			
• Transfusion reaction	• Septic thrombo-phlebitis			

Diagnosis

Review the details of the operation. The length of the operative time, estimated blood loss, use of preoperative antibiotics, concurrent medical problems, parity, and obesity can be risk factors for postoperative pyrexia. Take a detailed history and perform a systems review.

- *Atelectasis*: usually precedes pneumonia. Fever associated with this resolves following reinflation of the lungs. At risk are those with advanced age, obesity, current smoking habit, and a pre-existing chronic pulmonary disease.
- *Pneumonia*: 80% will have symptoms—cough, dyspnea, pleuritic chest pain, and purulent or blood-stained sputum.
- *Aspiration pneumonitis*: dyspnea, tachypnea, noisy respirations, and cough. Bacterial pneumonia will ensue in 50%.
- *Urinary tract infection*: if voiding freely, will have dysuria. May also be catheter-related.
- *Intraabdominal abscess*: complains of abdominal or pelvic pain.

Perform a thorough physical examination.

- *Atelectasis*: diminished breath sounds, percussive dullness, and elevation of the diaphragm over the affected side.
- *Pneumonia*: similar to atelectasis.

- Aspiration pneumonitis: tachypnea, chest wall retraction, bronchorrhea and bronchoconstriciton.
- Thrombophlebitis: non-infective—usually at IV infusion site. Common in patients with prolonged IV infusion or locally noxious drugs. May have superimposed bacterial contamination.
- Wound infection: inspect the wound. May be swollen, red, and indurated. May be expressing pus.
- Deep venous thrombosis: calf tenderness and swelling. Presence of Homans' sign (calf pain on dorsiflexion of the foot). Phlegmasia cerulean dolens (painful blue leg) is an extreme sign present in < 50% of cases.
- Intraabdominal abscess: tenderness on palpation. If sealed off, may present as a lump on palpation.

Investigations based on likely diagnosis.
- Pneumonia: chest X-ray. Sputum samples for Gram-stain smear. Cultures should also be obtained.
- Aspiration pneumonitis. chest X-ray.
- Wound infection: wound swab for bacterial culture or perform needle aspiration using aseptic technique.
- Urinary tract infection. urinalysis or MSU for culture and sensitivity.
- Deep venous thrombosis: venography is the standard means of diagnosis. Doppler ultrasonography is non-invasive and has a sensitivity and specificity of > 90%.
- Ultrasonography: collection of pus in the pelvis or subphrenic area. May mimic pleural effusion on a chest X-ray.

Management
- Atelectasis: if has any of these risk factors use bronchodilator therapy, including theophylline. Adequate analgesia. Incentive spirometry. Coughing to mobilize secretions. If still unsuccessful and if with extensive lobar collapse, flexible bronchoscopic aspiration is indicated. Secretions may be rendered less adherent by maintaining hydration and administering humidified air or oxygen and nebulized mucolytic agents. Once developed, coughing, deep breathing and incentive spirometry should be continued with greater intensity. Significant hypoxemia (PaO_2 <60 mmHg) should be corrected with oxygen therapy. Manoeuvers discussed above for clearance of secretions necessary. Drainage of pleural fluid or air via tube thoracostomy may be necessary to relieve compressive atelectasis.
- Pneumonia: organisms predominantly Gram-negative in nosocomial pneumonias. Includes Pseudomonas aeruginosa, Proteus mirabilis, Serratia marcescens, Escherichia coli, Klebsiella pneumoniae, and Enterobacter species. Staphylococcus aureus and Streptococcus pneumoniae in 14%. Anaerobic organisms in 2% and usually in aspiration pneumonia. Fungal uncommon. Supplemental oxygen. If severely compromised, require intubation and mechanical support. Begin empiric treatment: usually aminoglycoside and antipseudomonal penicillin. Antibiotic selection modified based on Gram-stain smear results. Culture results will guide more specific therapy.

- *Aspiration pneumonitis:* cases with distal airway obstruction evident on chest film will need flexible bronchoscopic aspiration of debris. Brochodilators necessary. If acute respiratory failure develops, postitive pressure ventilation.
- *Thrombophlebitis:* remove venous catheters. If bacterial contamination, treat with antibiotics. If suppurative, affected vein should be excised.
- *Wound infection:* oral or IV antibiotics and appropriate wound care. If wound collection present drainage should be performed. If systemically unwell or cellulitus may require IV antibiotics. If rapidly expanding or patches of skin necrosis at different sites, consider necrotizing fasciitis.
- *Urinary tract infection:* if urinalysis is positive, may start on empiric treatment. This may later be changed once sensitivity results are obtained.
- *Deep venous thrombosis:* prophylaxis is more important which includes wearing of pneumatic stockings and early mobilization. Use of anti-coagulants perioperatively is controversial. Treated with warfarin or fragmin.
- *Intra-abdominal abscess:* start empiric treatment with antibiotics. May require drainage.

Reference

1. Shwandt A, Andrews SJ, Fanning J (2001). Prospective analysis of a fever evaluation algorithm after major gynecologic surgery. *Am J Obstet Gynecol*, **184**, 1066–7.

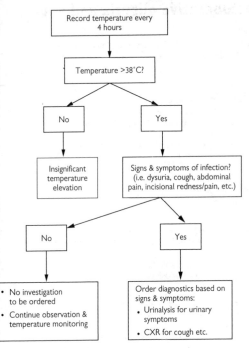

Fig. 11.1 Management algorithm[1]

☼ Postoperative oliguria and anuria

Definition
- *Oliguria*: urine output of <0.5 ml/kg/hr or <500 ml per 24 hr.
- *Anuria*: total absence of urinary excretion.

Causes
Pre-renal
- Hypovolemia secondary to:
  - intra or post-operative bleeding
  - inadequate intra-operative fluid administration
- Third space losses:
  - loss to extracellular space due to tissue damage
  - cardiac failure
  - pulmonary oedema
- Cardiac suppression:
  - anaesthetic agents
  - elderly.

Renal
- Acute renal failure e.g. acute tubular necrosis secondary to haemorrhage
- Acute on chronic renal failure e.g. exacerbation of underlying renal disease
- Nephrotoxicity of anaesthetic agents
- Other drugs e.g. aminoglycosides

Post-renal
- Blocked urinary catheter (debris, blood, clamped, or kinked catheter)
- Urinary retention (infection, frank haematuria, oedema, or haematoma at bladder base)
- Unrecognized bladder perforation (laparoscopy, CS, cystoscopy)
- Ureteric injury or obstruction (transection, ligation, kinking, spasm, oedema)*
- Urethral injury or obstruction*
- Vulval, vaginal or paraurethral haematoma
- Pain.

Management
Initial steps
- Check pulse and BP to determine urgency of problem
- Exclude intra-abdominal or vaginal bleeding
- Read operative notes if not personally involved in surgery
- Check fluid-balance chart and ensure adequate intake
- Exclude obstructed catheter
- Try to determine cause (pre-renal, renal, post-renal).

Surgical procedures that may give rise to the above complications
- Incontinence surgery (colposuspension, tape suspension procedures)
- Prolapse surgery (procidentia)
- Complex abdominal hysterectomy (fibroids, endometriosis)
- Complicated CS (haemorrhage, full dilatation, Caesarean hysterectomy)

Pre-renal and renal cause
- Exclude pulmonary oedema and congestive cardiac failure (basal crackles, tachypnea, raised JVP)
- Fluid challenge of 400 ml crystalloid (normal saline, Hartmann's solution)(colloids e.g. Gelofusine®, Haemacell® are expensive and can cause anaphylaxis)
- Expect response of at least 30 ml/hr
- Attempt second fluid challenge
- Liaise with anaesthetist and physician
- Consider IV frusemide
- If no response insert CVP line
  - if CVP low give more fluid
  - if CVP high give frusemide.
- Aim for CVP of 0–6 mmHg
- Consider transfer to ITU

Post-renal

Acute retention
- Pass a urethral or suprapubic indwelling catheter—leave on free drainage 24–48 hours
- Treat infection

Obstructed catheter
- If catheter is obstructed, flush bladder or replace with larger catheter (especially with frank haematuria)
- Consider cause of bleeding
- Consider double or triple lumen catheter and regular bladder flushing with large clots
- Consider antibiotics

Ureteric injury
- Signs—loin pain, uraemia (NB—sometimes there is no pain)
- Do not give fluid challenge
- U&E, ABG if uraemic
- Ultrasound for hydronephrosis determine level of obstruction
- Refer to urogynaecology or urology immediately if confirmed.

Return to theatre
- Cystourethroscopy
- Ureteric catheterization and retrograde pyelogram to detemine type and level of obstruction.

Management options
- Removal of suture
- Reimplantation of ureter
- Defunctioning nephrostomy.

Failure to recognize and treat may be associated with permanent renal impairment.

Chapter 12

Ovarian hyperstimulation syndrome

Kamal Ojha

⊕ Ovarian hyperstimulation syndrome

Ovarian hyperstimulation syndrome (OHSS) is the most serious complication of ovulation induction. With the introduction of gonadotrophin-releasing hormone (GnRH) agonists and the use of higher doses of menotrophins to retrieve a higher number of mature oocytes to maximize ART pregnancy rates, the incidence of severe OHSS has increased. After in vitro fertilization (IVF) and embryo transfer, the overall incidence of OHSS is reported to be 0.6–14%; however, the incidence of severe OHSS is ~1–2%.

The pathogenesis of OHSS is still unclear. It has been suggested that, in the presence of high concentrations of oestrogen, there is an increase in capillary permeability, which leads to a shift of fluid to the extravascular compartments (mainly the peritoneal cavity) with the formation of ascites.

- Mild cases of OHSS are characterized by the formation of multiple ovarian cysts associated with excess steroid production and ovarian enlargement.
- Moderate OHSS is associated with abdominal distention, nausea, diarrhoea or vomiting.
- In severe OHSS, ascites, hydrothorax, electrolyte imbalance, haemo-concentration, hypovolaemia, oliguria, or thromboemboli have been reported. This could be fatal if not treated promptly.

Management

The management of mild and moderate OHSS is expectant, while the management of severe forms of OHSS includes hospitalization for fluid and electrolyte management, paracentesis, or continuous drainage of the ascitic fluid if necessary[1] and mini-dose heparin prophylaxis to prevent thromboembolic complications[2]. IV albumin is given to retain fluid in the intravascular compartment. Close monitoring with FBC, U&E, LFTs and clotting profile is the key to management.

Prevention of OHSS

Individualizing ovulation induction protocols for each patient according to different variables may lead to a better control of ovarian hyperstimulation.

Factors which increase the risk of OHSS are:
- Age of the patient (younger patients are at higher risk)
- Weight (thin-built are more at risk)
- Day 3 serum follicle stimulating hormone (lower levels)
- A history of exaggerated response in previous induction of ovulation cycles.
- Patients with polycystic ovary syndrome or who have a sonographic appearance of multicystic ovaries at baseline ultrasound evaluation.

The above group is at risk for developing OHSS and should be treated less aggressively with menotrophins.

OHSS can be avoided by not administering HCG, and aborting the cycle in patients who have a serum oestradiol concentration of >10 000 pmol/L or who have >20 follicles seen on ultrasound before oocyte retrieval, especially if most of the follicles have the mean follicular diameter <12 mm. Although this is a good preventive measure for avoiding OHSS, it is frustrating for both the patient and the treating physician.

Using progesterone rather than HCG for luteal phase support has also been suggested in patients who are at risk of developing OHSS. Withholding HCG and menotrophins for a number of days called 'coasting', while continuing GnRH agonists until serum oestradiol concentrations return to a reasonable value (<10 000 pmol/L), has been widely used and is successful in preventing OHSS. This strategy shows no deleterious effect on the oocyte quality or on pregnancy rate.

Cryopreserving all embryos and transferring them later in another cycle has been used as another way of avoiding OHSS[3]. Some authors have reported that the administration of IV albumin during or after oocyte retrieval prevents OHSS. However, most of the later reports have shown that IV administration of albumin does not help in preventing OHSS[4].

References

1. Al-Ramahi M, Leader A, Claman P et al. (1997). A novel approach to the treatment of ascites associated with ovarian hyperstimulation syndrome. Hum Reprod, **12**, 2614–16.
2. Hignett M, Spence JEH, Claman P (1995). Internal jugular vein thrombosis: a late complication of ovarian hyper stimulation syndrome despite mini-dose heparin prophylaxis. Hum Reprod, **10**, 3121–3.
3. Tiitinen A, Husa LM, Tulppala M, et al. (1995). The effect of cryopreservation in prevention of ovarian hyperstimulation syndrome. Br J Obstet Gynaecol, **102**(4), 326–9.
4. Rizk B (1999). Ovarian hyperstimulation syndrome. In PR Brindsen, and PA Rainsbury (eds), The Bourn Hall Textbook of In vitro Fertilization and Assisted Conception, 2nd edition, Parthenon, London, pp. 369–3.

Contraception and termination of pregnancy

Penny Oakeley

Kamal Ojha

⊘ Unprotected intercourse (emergency contraception)

Risk of unwanted pregnancy after sexual intercourse without adequate contraceptive precautions.

Definition of inadequate contraception

- No contraception
- Unreliable method used—e.g. coitus interruptus
- Reliable method used incorrectly:
  - slipped or broken condom
  - displaced diaphragm or cap within 6 hours of intercourse
  - partially expelled IUCD or IUCD removal with history of intercourse in previous 7 days
  - late starting new packet of combined oral contraception
  - pills taken over 12 hours late in days 1–7 of a new pack
  - more than 4 consecutive missed pills in days 8–14 of pack
  - missed pills in days 15–21 *do not* require EC if the next packet is started without the pill-free interval of 7 days (i.e. she takes 2 packets consecutively)
- Over 3 hours late with older progestogen-only pills (Cerazette® allows 12 hours)
- Over 14 weeks since last Depo-Provera® injection

Types of emergency contraception

- Hormonal (EHC)
  - Levonelle®-2 (progestogen-only)
  - PC4 (combined oral) *no longer available*
  - Mifepristone *not available for this use in the UK*
- Copper-bearing IUCD

Presentation and management

- If < 72 hr (3 days) emergency hormonal contraception (EHC) may be administered: a stat dose of levonorgestrel tabs 150 µg (Levonelle × 2). Exclude the possibility of existing pregnancy or previous unprotected sexual intercourse (UPSI) > 72 hours previously. Unlicensed use may be up to 120 hr (5 days).
- There is no limit to the number of times EHC may be given in a cycle. It will not harm a fetus if it has failed.
- Consider a copper IUCD if the woman is at ovulation (levonorgestrel may only act by postponing or abolishing ovulation but a copper IUCD will prevent implantation). *Do not use a hormone-bearing IUCD or IUS.*
- If she is < 120 hours of UPSI, a copper-bearing IUCD may be inserted after a single UPSI at any time of the cycle.
- A copper-bearing IUCD may be fitted up to 5 days after presumed ovulation in a regular cycle (day 19 of a 28 day cycle), however, many episodes of UPSI have taken place.

Important considerations

- Always consider future contraception and advise restarting the chosen method immediately with precautions for 7 days. Starting oral contraception immediately will not harm a fetus if EHC fails.[2]
- Some people advise giving Depo-Provera immediately. The patient should ideally abstain totally from intercourse for 48 hours and have a pregnancy test in 3–4 weeks time.
- If an emergency copper IUCD is inserted, but the woman wishes to use an alternative method after her next period, provide her with her alternative to start with the next cycle before removal of the device.
- Consider screening for sexually transmitted infections or referral to genito-urinary medicine if the sexual intercourse was casual or forced. Refer early for forensic tests after rape, if the patient agrees.
- Where the girl is under 16 or suffering from learning disability or mental health problems, consider competence to consent to future contraception (Fraser Guidelines—see box). EC should not be withheld however.
- Pre-pubertal girls do not need EC, although it is possible to conceive before the first menses.
- Postmenopausal women over 50 do not need EC, if there have been no periods for 12 months (2 years if under 50). Women on HRT may need EC.
- Women taking interacting medication such as some anti-epileptics should take 2 Levonelle tabs stat and repeat the dose in 12 hrs.

Fraser Guidelines

Competence to consent to contraception

For a girl under 16 to consent to contraception advice or treatment the guidelines, laid down by Lord Fraser in the House of Lords (1985) require the professional to be satisfied:

1) That she understands the advice
2) That she cannot be persuaded to inform her parents or allow the doctor to inform her parents
3) That she will continue to have sexual intercourse ± contraception
4) That her physical or mental health (or both) is likely to suffer unless she receives contraception advice or treatment
5) That it is in the best interests of the girl to receive contraception advice or treatment (or both) without parental consent

Consider the possibility of sexual abuse, especially if the age gap is more than 3 years. It is an absolute offence for a man to have intercourse with a girl under the age of 13. All cases of children under the age of 13 believed to be engaged in penetrative sexual relationships or activity must be referred to Children's Social Services and the Police (Sexual Offences Act 2003).

Further Reading

1. von Hertzen H, Piaggio G, Ding J, et al. (2002). Low dose mifepristone and two regimens of levonorgestrel for emergency contraception. *Lancet*, **360**, 1803–10.
2. Kubba A, Sanfilippo J, Hampton N (eds) (1999). *Contraception and Office Gynaecology*. W.B. Saunders, Philadelphia.
3. Durand M, del Carmen Cravioto M, Raymond EG, et al. (2001). On the mechanisms of action of short-lived levonorgestrel administration in emergency contraception. *Contraception*, **64**, 227–34.
4. Webb A (2003). Emergency contraception. *BMJ*, **326**, 775–6.
5. Faculty of Family Planning and Reproductive Health Care of the RCOG Guidance www.ffprhc.org.uk.

:⊙: Complications associated with termination of pregnancy

Abortion is one of the commonest gynaecological procedures performed all over the world. In the UK 186 000 abortions were performed in England and Wales, and 12 000 in Scotland in the late 1990s.

Complications of abortion can cause significant morbidity. Fortunately mortality is low in the UK. Complications of abortion can be broadly grouped under 3 categories.

- Procedure related complications
- Psychological complications
- Anaesthesia related complications.

Procedure-related complications

The complications depend upon the method of TOP, which can be medical or surgical.

Uterine perforation

- The plastic cannula or the cervical dilator used during surgical TOP may perforate the uterus. The risk is very low with an experienced surgeon and is increased with previous surgery on the uterus and increasing period of gestation. The risk reported is 1–4 per 1000. Uterine perforation can become a life-threatening complication due to severe haemorrhage and damage to the intraperitoneal contents, especially the bowel.
- If perforation is suspected the vacuum in the cannula should be broken before withdrawing the cannula and a laparoscopy performed to assess bleeding and to safely evacuate the products of conception.
- The laparoscopy also helps in assessing the uterus and bowel. A laparotomy may be required to maintain haemostasis or repair of bowel.
- Perforation of the uterus can also injure the bladder and result in suprapubic pain and haematuria.
- Early detection and treatment will result in a good outcome.

Injury to cervix

Laceration of the cervix can happen due to rapid dilation of the cervix as done in surgical TOP. Cervical priming with a prostaglandin (misoprostol) transvaginally, usually 3 hours before the procedure can minimise this complication.

Haemorrhage

Excessive haemorrhage during or after abortion may signify uterine atony, cervical laceration, uterine perforation, cervical pregnancy, or coagulopathy. Haemorrhage can be severe enough to necessitate blood transfusion with the attendant risks of transfusion. The risk of haemorrhage following surgical TOP is around 1/1000 overall; it is 0.88 for gestation < 13 weeks and 4/1000 after 20 wk gestation.

Incomplete abortion

- This occurs due to some of the products of conception remaining inside the uterus after the abortion procedure is over. 5 per cent of women undergoing TOP will require surgical evacuation within the first month. It is more common as the period of gestation increases.

- The patient presents a few days after the TOP with persistent bleeding, heavy bleeding, or both. They can also present with features of infection, i.e. dull and/or colicky lower abdominal pain and low grade fever.
- The combination of pain, fever and bleeding is known as the post-abortion triad. An ultrasound of the uterus helps in diagnosis and in making the decision regarding evacuating the products of conception. However, blood clots in the uterus may make ultrasound diagnosis of retained products unreliable in these cases. In the presence of continued bleeding or symptoms and signs of infection, careful evacuation of the uterus may be needed.

Infection

- 1 per cent of women develop infection following TOP. This could be due to exacerbation of an underlying infection, not uncommon in sexually active women, introduction of infection during the procedures, or retained products of conception, which acts as a culture media for the organisms.
- If infection is not treated, it may lead to chronic pelvic inflammatory disease and infertility. Hence all women undergoing TOP should be offered prophylactic broad-spectrum antibiotics usually combination of doxycycline and metronidazole.

Vasovagal syncope

Vasovagal syncope may occur due to rapid dilation of the cervix. Recovery is the rule. This is not a feature when the procedure is done under good spinal or general anaesthetic.

Failed abortion

Failure to terminate pregnancy is greater with very early abortions (<6 wk gestational age). Such patients may present with symptoms of continuing pregnancy such as hyperemesis, increased abdominal girth, and breast engorgement. The failure rate is 2.3 per 1000 for surgical abortion and 1 to 14 per 1000 in medical abortion. Post termination follow-up 2 weeks after the procedure, a urine pregnancy test, and an ultrasound scan in suspected cases of failed abortion is practiced in some centres.

DIC

Suspect DIC in all patients who present with severe post-abortion bleeding, especially after mid-trimester abortions. Incidence is approximately 200/100 000 abortions; this rate is even higher for saline instillation techniques which is rarely required. This is a possible complication of evacuation of missed miscarriage >4 weeks.

Infertility

Rarely, abortion can result in infertility due to tubal block resulting from infection or due to vigorous curettage resulting in Ashermann's syndrome.

Future pregnancy

There is no evidence to support the risk of infertility, ectopic pregnancy, placenta previa, cervical incompetence, and pre-term delivery after TOPs. Prophylactive antibiotics and cervical priming with prostaglandins has helped in the prevention of these complications.

Anaesthesia-related complications

Most women prefer GA and it is generally safe. However, the risk of GA is increased in women > 35 years of age, increased BMI, heavy smokers, hypertension, cardiac and respiratory disease. If local anaesthesia is used, which is usually in the form of paracervical block, the complication due to inadvertent injection of the drug into the vessels can be life threatening leading to convulsion and cardiopulmonary arrest.

Psychological complications

Many women feel tearful and emotional for few days after an abortion. However, most of them recover. There is no risk of developing serious psychiatric illness because of abortion. There may be life-style factors that may influence how women feel after an abortion.

Vaginal discharge

Kamal Ojha

⑦ Abnormal vaginal discharge

Vaginal discharge can be physiological or pathological. Physiological discharge occurs during ovulation, premenstrually, pregnancy, and sexual stimulation. Pathological discharge is differentiated from physiological discharge by the presence of foul smell, blood staining, or pruritus. Abnormal vaginal discharge is one of the common symptoms encountered in the gynaecology clinic.

The causes are mostly infective in the reproductive age group and mostly non-infective in the postmenopausal age group.

Common causes

- Inflammation of the vagina also called vaginitis (most common)
- Pelvic inflammatory disease
- Tumours—both benign and malignant
- Atrophy of the vagina
- Foreign body—IUD, tampon
- Allergy to chemicals.

Inflammation of the vagina

Bacterial vaginosis, vaginal candidiasis, and *Trichomonas vaginalis* infection are thought to cause approximately 90 per cent of all vaginal infections. Bacterial vaginosis is the most common cause of vaginitis, accounting for 50 per cent of vaginitis cases. A thorough history and vaginal examination followed by bacteriological tests will help in the diagnosis.

- Bacterial vaginosis is diagnosed by thin white-grey discharge, vaginal pH >4.5, clue cells, and whiff test on KOH wet mount.
- Candidiasis is characterized by presence of erythema and adherent thick cottage cheese-like discharge.
- *Trichomonas vaginalis* infection is characterized by erythema, presence of a homogenous discharge, which may be green in colour, and strawberry appearance of the cervix.

Pelvic inflammatory disease

Inflammation of the cervix, uterus, and tubes can cause abnormal vaginal discharge, which is most commonly caused by sexually acquired infections of which *Chlamydia trachomatis* and *Neisseria gonorrhoeae* are the common ones. Abdominal pain, pain during intercourse and during bimanual vaginal examination is usually present.

Tumours

Both benign and malignant tumour of the vulva, vagina, cervix, and uterus can cause abnormal vaginal discharge. The most common benign tumour in the uterus is fibroid and is most likely to cause vaginal discharge if it is a submucosal or a fibroid polyp protruding through the cervical canal. Malignant lesion of the cervix and the uterus also cause vaginal discharge. Post-coital or contact bleeding may indicate a cervical lesion that may be malignant or pre-malignant.

Atrophy of the vaginal epithelium

Menopausal changes in the vagina predispose it to the inflammatory process and can result in abnormal vaginal discharge. However, abnormal vaginal discharge in postmenopausal women should prompt a search for a malignant cause before considering vaginal atrophy as a cause.

Foreign body

Any foreign body in the genital tract will evoke an inflammatory response and lead to discharge from the vagina. Forgotten tampons in the vagina can cause offensive vaginal discharge. IUDs may produce vaginal discharge although not severe.

Allergy to chemicals

The chemicals used in personal hygiene products can cause allergy and produce inflammation of the vulva and vagina.

History

Time pattern

- When did this begin?
- Does the discharge remain constant throughout the month?

Quality

- What does the discharge look like (colour and consistency)?
- Is there an odour?
- Is there pain, itching, or burning?

Aggravating factors

- Does sexual intercourse increase the symptoms?
- Does your sexual partner have a penile discharge?
- Do you have multiple sexual partners or sexual partners that you do not know very well?

Relieving factors

- Is there anything that relieves the discharge?
- Does frequent bathing help?
- Have over-the-counter creams been tried?
- Has douching been tried? What kind?

What other symptoms are present?

- Abdominal pain?
- Vaginal itching?
- Fever?
- Vaginal bleeding?
- Rash?
- Warts?
- Other lesions?
- Changes in urination?
- Difficulty or pain on urination?
- Blood in urine?
- Diarrhoea?

Other important information
- What medications are being taken?
- What is the frequency of sexual activity?
- Do you use condoms?
- Do you have any allergies?
- Have you changed the detergents or soaps that you use?
- Do you frequently wear very tight pants?

Investigations

- MSU, high vaginal and endocervical swabs for culture and sensitivity.
- FBC, U&Es, LFTs.
- Urinary pregnancy test to exclude pregnancy.
- Pelvic utrasound for benign lesions and pelvic collection.

Treatment

The treatment of infective pathology is briefly discussed in this section.
- Removal of foreign body and IUCD before initiating treatment is essential.
- Antibiotics and anti-inflammatory agents need to be started after the swabs and bloods have been performed.
- Chlamydia—doxycycline 100 mg bd for 7 days is the first line of choice. Azithromycin and erythromycin can also be used.
- Bacterial vaginosis—metronidazole 400 mg orally bd for 7 days. IV or PR routes may be necessary .
- Candidiasis—clotrimazole 500 mg daily intravaginally for 7 days.

In severe cases, especially in those with pelvic inflammatory disease, IV antibiotics may need to be prescribed. Diagnostic laparoscopy may be required if symptoms do not resolve within 24–48 hr.

Long term effects
The most deleterious effect of pelvic infection is the possibility of tubal damage. Urgent investigations and early treatment even prior to receiving the results is needed to prevent tubal damage.

Non-infective causes are discussed with postmenopausal discharge.

⑦ Peri- and postmenopausal discharge

Discharge occurring per vaginum in older women has different causes and merits separate attention from those occurring in younger women. Perimenopause is defined as the period, occurring few years before the onset of menopause during which the woman is going through the menopausal change. The main concern of vaginal discharge in perimenopausal and postmenopausal women is that it could be a harbinger of malignant change in the genital tract, as genital tract malignancy is much higher in this age group. Hence any abnormal vaginal discharge in the perimenopausal women and any discharge in the postmenopausal women warrant immediate evaluation.

Causes
- Endometrial carcinoma
- Cervical carcinoma
- Hormone replacement therapy
- Endometrial hyperplasia
- Endometrial polyp
- Fibroid uterus
- Endometrial atrophy
- Atophic vaginitis
- Vaginal pessaries
- Foreign bodies—IUD
- Vaginal and vulval carcinoma
- Infectious causes—candidiasis.

Of all the above causes, benign causes are more common than the malignant ones. But the approach towards the patient would be to rule out the malignant causes before proceeding with the treatment.

A complete history should be obtained especially with regard to the onset, duration, severity of the symptoms, use of HRT, use of tamoxifen, and history of cervical smears.

In postmenopausal women, the most common causes of bleeding or blood-stained discharge are benign conditions (88 per cent) of which atrophic vaginitis is the most common. Up to 12 per cent of the women may have a malignant condition of which the most common is endometrial carcinoma. Hence, in managing postmenopausal women with bleeding or discharge, an active search for malignancy is warranted. This is accomplished by a speculum examination for cervical lesions, performing a transvaginal scan, and a pipelle endometrial biopsy.

Atrophic vaginitis is due to lack of oestrogen in menopause and hence application of oestrogen cream in the vagina will relieve the symptoms.

In the perimenopausal women, malignancy may be a possibility and the first priority is to rule out malignancy before proceeding with the treatment. A pelvic examination, transvaginal ultrasound, endometrial sampling are basic requirements to rule out malignant disease in the genital tract. A hysteroscopy and curettage is a definitive diagnostic procedure. The treatment depends on the particular diagnosis.

Vulval problems

Sarah Harper and David Nunns

⑦ Pruritus vulvae/vulvodynia

Pruritus vulvae

Differential diagnosis
- Lichen sclerosus
- Lichen simplex
- Contact dermatitis
- Psoriasis
- Infection
- Lichen planus.

Lichen sclerosus
Autoimmune inflammatory condition of skin. Mainly affecting the genital area in women.
- Diagnosis
  - white, crinkly skin, anatomy of vulva lost and labial adhesions.
  - rubbing of skin causes thickened lichenified areas.
  - histological biopsy to confirm diagnosis in difficult cases.
- Treatment
  - dermovate ointment (clobetasol propionate 0.05 per cent) is applied bd for 8 wk.
  - continued with maintenance dose usually 1–2 per week
  - lower dose steroid creams often not effective
  - emollients, E45® and aqueous cream can be helpful.
  - surgery to divide adhesions at fouchette may be needed.
  - need follow-up as risk of vulval cancer developing (<5% risk).

Lichen simplex
- Diagnosis
Lichenified skin secondary to scratching. Often psychosomatic and sometimes unilateral on side of dominant hand.
- Treatment
Use Dermovate® ointment to control situation using same dosing regime as lichen sclerosis. Atarax® (hydroxyzine hydrochloride) 25 mg at night may be useful to control pruritis. Can increase up to tds until relief. Hygiene, counselling, and support very important.

Contact dermatitis
- Diagnosis
Take a careful history to try to identify irritant. On examination often red and swollen with possible evidence of secondary infection.
- Treatment
  - Eliminate irritant, try 1 per cent hydrocortisone cream for relief of symptoms and possible antibiotics if secondary infection.
  - Advise on avoiding perfumed products and aqueous cream for washing.

Psoriasis
- Diagnosis

Unusual for first presentation to be on vulva, characteristic scaling patches not often seen.
  - For treatment try moderately potent topical steroid.
  - Refer to specialist vulval/dermatology clinic.

Infection
- Diagnosis

Consider referral to GUM clinic if sexually transmitted disease suspected.
- Treatment

Common cause Candida, associated with thick white discharge can be treated with antifungal pessary clotrimazole 50 mg once at night ± topical cream.

Lichen planus
- Diagnosis
  - Purple/white papules, can affect any area of body. Usually self-limiting and often asymptomatic.
  - Histological biopsy will confirm diagnosis.
- Treatment

Try treating with Dermovate® ointment if symptomatic.

General considerations for good practice
- When prescribing steroids be specific about dose e.g. Dermovate® 0.5 g or pea-sized amount applied bd to affected skin for 8 wk.
- Need to massage into affected skin areas.
- Ointments are less irritant than creams.
- Irritability from topical agents is common on vulval skin.
- Emollients e.g. E45®/aqueous cream are bland and scent free, very useful for soothing and rehydrating dry inflammed skin.
- Good hygiene is essential, use aqueous cream as soap substitute.
- Biopsy can be very useful in difficult cases.

Vulvodynia
Burning or soreness of the vulva in the absence of infection or a dermatological cause.

Causes
- Unknown
- Neurogenic pain.

Acute causes resulting in nerve injury pain are rare
- Spinal cord injury
- Meningeal cyst.

Presentation
- Variable age group.
- Constant pain 'unprovoked vulvodynia'
- Pain on light touch 'provoked vulvodynia' results in dysparenuria. Formerly vestibulitus.
- Often nothing to see on vulva, sore spots with provoked vulvodynia.

Diagnosis
- Clinical diagnosis, no need for biopsies.

Treatment
- Support and reassurance are important.
- Address neuropathic pain, using tricyclic antidepressants which at low doses have analgesic properties. Amitriptyline can be commenced, 10 mg at night and increased by 10 mg daily until pain-free, on average this will take 60–100 mg daily. (Max 150 mg per day.) Usually 3 month course will be adequate, side-effects can be difficult to tolerate.
- As a second line, neuroleptics such as gabapentin may be of benefit.
- Local anaesthetic gels e.g. lignocaine 1–2% may be applied to reduce skin sensitivity. (10% may have irritation after application.)
- Good hygiene—wash only with water and avoid scented products.
- Consider referral to vulval clinic for difficult cases, rarely surgery may be indicated for provoked vulvodynia.

⑦ **Lump or ulcer at vulva**

Vulval lumps

Malignant

- Uncommon, incidence approx 3:100 000
- Often in older age group, need urgent outpatient referral.

Differential diagnosis

1. Squamous cell carcinoma
2. Melanoma
3. Bartholin's gland
4. Basal cell carcinoma
5. Verrucous

- 85 per cent squamous cell, often complain of a mass and itching, less often discharge and bleeding.
- Diagnosis confirmed with histological biopsy, important to palpate inguinal nodes.
- 5 per cent melanoma, can present complaining of an enlarged mole, prognosis is dependent on depth of invasion. Mainstay of treatment surgical, vulval skin prone to desquamation with radiotherapy.
- 10 per cent made up of other causes, all very rare would need urgent biopsy for histological diagnosis.
- Refer all cases to gynaeoncology team.

Benign

Common.

Differential diagnosis

- Bartholin's gland
- Ectopic tissue (e.g. endometrioma)
- Lipomas/fibroma
- Squamous papillomata 'skin tag'
- Folliculitis—infected hair follicle
- Condyloma acuminata 'warts'
- Many others usually diagnosed histologically.

Bartholin's abscess or cyst

- Gland situated in posterior 1/3 of labia majora and lower vagina.
- Abscess will be very painful. Antibiotics can be used flucloxacillin 500 mg qid but often need acute referral for incision and drainage. Marsupialisation is performed to help prevent recurrence.
- Send pus swab for culture. Can be associated with gonorrheoa. Useful to check blood glucose.

Ectopic tissue

Usually histological diagnosis, think of breast tissue if presents or increases in size in pregnancy, or endometriosis if cyclical nature to mass.

Skin tags
Very common, be reassuring, only refer or treat if symptomatic. May often be excised under local anaesthetic.

Condyloma acuminata
- Common finding, associated with human papilloma virus (HPV) 6 and 11.
- Diagnosis is clinical but can be confirmed with biopsy.
- Contact tracing is necessary so refer to GUM clinic.
- Treatment is usually with topical podophyllin, cryotherapy, or surgery.

Vulval ulcer
Differential diagnosis
- Herpes
- Apthous ulcers
- Syphyllis
- Vulval carcinoma
- Crohn's disease
- Bechet's disease

Herpes
- Viral origin, in UK 50% herpes simplex II 'cold sores'
- Incubation period 2–14 days, primary attack can be severe lasting 3–4 wk if not treated. Recurrent attacks shorter and less severe.
- Essential to refer to GUM clinic for contact tracing and screening for other infections.
- Usually present with painful ulcerated vulva, possible intact vesicles.
- Associated with fever, malaise and possible inguinal lymphadenopathy.
- Diagnosis is clinical but vesicular fluid can be sent for viral culture.
- Treatment comprises of rest and analgesia, Aciclovir may be effective to limit severity and duration. Use 200 mg five times daily for 5 days.
- Consider suprapubic catheter if patient presents with urinary retention.

Apthous ulcer
- Analogous to mouth ulcer, small and painful with a yellow base, usually labia majora not associated with systemic upset.
- Simple pain relief, self limiting.

Syphyllis
- Indurated painless 'chancre', can be on vulva or cervix, may have several.
- Refer to GUM clinic for treatment and contact tracing.

Crohn's disease
- Up to 30 per cent of sufferers may have vulval involvement, can preceed GI involvement. Appear like knife cuts to skin.
- If there is already GI involvement, look for sinuses and discharge.

Bechet's disease
- Chronic picture, can also affect mouth and eyes.
- Can last for months, no specific histological changes to aid diagnosis.

Miscellaneous topics in gynaecology

Michelle Fynes

**Rukma Bhattacharya and
Sambit Mukhopadhyay**

⚙ Urinary retention

Definitions
- Acute retention: sudden onset of painful or painless inability to void over 12 hours, requiring catheterization with removal of a volume equal to or greater than normal bladder capacity.
- Chronic retention: insidious and painless failure of bladder emptying where catheterization yields a volume equal to at least 50 per cent of normal bladder capacity.

Signs and symptoms
- Pain
- Overflow incontinence
- Frequency
- Poor flow
- Intermittent stream
- Incomplete emptying
- Straining to void
- Hesitancy
- Palpable bladder, dull to percussion.

Causes of

Neurological disease
- As a result of spinal injury—spinal shock phase
- Upper motor neuron lesion—spinal injury, multiple sclerosis
- Lower motor neuron lesion—spinal injury, multiple sclerosis
- Autonomic lesion e.g. after pelvic surgery
- Local pain reflex after surgery.

Pharmacological
- Tricyclic antidepressants, anticholinergic agents
- α-adrenergic agents, epidural, and spinal anaesthesia.

Acute Inflammation
- Acute urethritis, acute cystitis, acute vulvovaginitis
- Acute anogenital infection.

Obstruction
- Distal urethral stenosis, acute urethral oedema after surgery
- Chronic urethral stenosis, foreign body or calculus in the urethra
- Distortion of urethra by cystocele or uterine prolapse
- Impacted pelvic mass (retroverted gravid uterus, haematocolpos, uterine fibroids, ovarian cyst, faecal impaction)
- Bladder leiomyoma

Endocrine
Hypothyroidism, diabetic neuropathy.

Overdistension
Post-surgical
- Surgery for stress incontinence, anorectal surgery
- Pelvic surgery (especially radical).

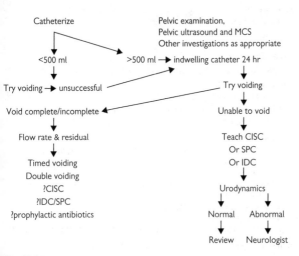

Fig. 16.1 Acute retention

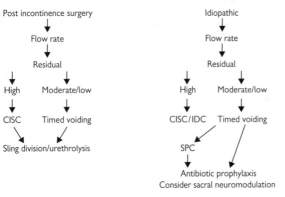

Fig. 16.2 Chronic retention

CISC: clean intermittent self-catheterization; IDC: indwelling urethral catheter; SPC: suprapubic catheter, MCS: microscopy, culture and sensitivity.

Psychogenic

Anxiety or depressive illness, hysteria

Idiopathic

Investigations

Investigations should be performed with the suspected abnormality in mind.

Acute retention

- Urine MCS and cytology in all cases
- Pass a urethral catheter to measure urinary volume and may leave on for free drainage.

Chronic retention

- Determine residual volume by post-micturition ultrasound or catheterization
- Uroflowmetry
  - maximum urinary flow rate (abnormal if <15 ml/sec for a void of at least 150 ml)
  - time to void may be delayed
  - prolonged voiding time
  - abnormal flow pattern (saw tooth appearance as straining to void).

Other investigations to be considered as appropriate

- U&E
- Pelvic and renal ultrasound
- Cystometrogram
- Lumbosacral spine X-ray, e.g. spina bifida and intervertabral disc prolapse
- Cystourethroscopy e.g. urethral stenosis or stricture, bladder diverticulae
- Electromyography e.g. urethral sphincter hypertrophy, multiple system atrophy.

Management

Exclude UTI in all cases.

✪ Sexual assault

Incidence

The lifetime risk of sexual assault is 1 in 4–6 for women but the incidence of child sexual abuse is unknown. 1 in 5 adult rapes are reported but probably only 1 in 20–50 assaults of children are known to supervising authorities. In the UK in 2004, 190 000 were victims of serious sexual assault and there were 47 000 female victims of rape or attempted rape. The definition of sexual offences and rape vary from country to country but the recent British Sexual Offences Act 2003[1] has sought to clarify the law with respect to current patterns of sexual violence and exploitation. In summary this act defines rape as any non-consensual penetration of the mouth, vagina, or anus by a penis. Sexual assault replaces indecent assault which is defined as penetration involving the insertion of an object, or body parts other than the penis, into the vagina or anus. Children under 13 cannot legally consent to sexual activity. Child sex offences include activity with no sexual contact (i.e. forcing child to watch sexual act). 'Familial child sex offences' replace 'incest' to incorporate the wider context of the modern family and includes non-blood relatives. Offences of abuse of trust is an abuse of children through prostitution (direct or indirect) and pornography/trafficking/grooming.

Risks of sexual assault

- 1 in 4–6 women lifetime risk
- 1 in 10 sexual assault of men-lifetime risk
- From reported sexual assaults data—12% by strangers, 45% acquaintances, 43% intimate partners
- When assessing a potential victim, it is important to establish whether a sexual act has occurred and whether they gave consent when they were competent to give consent.

Presentation

Acute or delayed or acute on chronic (particularly for children) presentation may occur.

Acute sexual assault

- 16–58% have genital injuries
- 38–80% have non-genital injuries
- May present to A&E or via the police
- May present to GU medicine/gynaecological/psychiatric services with covert or overt symptoms.

Delayed

- GU medicine
- Gynaecology
- Antenatally (increase in domestic violence and assault during pregnancy).

Concerns arising for children

- Repeated A&E attendances
- Poor parent–child interactions or behaviour

- Child known to social services
- Any injuries to child under 1 year
- Domestic abuse
- Explanation inconsistent with injuries
- Disclosure of abuse by child
- Delay in presentation

Management

Needs of the victim to be addressed are:
- Medical
- Psychological
- Forensic.

Immediate medical care is the first priority (this will determine the venue of examination).

- Appropriate therapeutic measures—this includes resuscitation and usual 'ABC' measures are of overriding importance irrespective of forensic evidence
  - bleeding
  - loss of consciousness (injury/intoxication)
  - oxygenation
- Consideration of collection of evidence (Locards principle 1928— 'every contact leaves a trace'—loss of 'best evidence' must be a consideration if someone wishes to have the option of forensic investigation)
- Prophylactic antibiotics
- Post exposure prophylaxis for HIV
- Emergency contraception
- Hepatitis B vaccination
- Analgesia
- General advice and support, follow-up including counselling.

Consideration of the presence of a responsible adult/carer for children or adults without mental capacity and interpreters must be considered before examination in non-life threatening situations. If impairment of capacity to consent to examination is temporary, for example due to drugs or alcohol, then an appropriate time and setting should be awaited.

Those > 16 are able to consent and children < 16 who are considered Fraser-competent do not need an adult present although this should be recommended by health care professionals. All forensic examinations of victims < 13 should occur with a trained examiner with a trained paediatrician.

In A&E departments there should be 'early evidence kits' where samples of urine and saliva can be taken before the victim decides whether to proceed with forensic investigation. This decreases the chance of loss or contamination of delicate evidence. In some units there may be provision of forensic swabs but the collection of forensic data requires a huge amount of documentation that if not properly undertaken may prove useless or even harmful to the case if brought to court. For these reasons these samples are ideally taken by trained professionals[2] or under close supervision. The police are usually able to provide further information if requested. In London, Manchester, and Newcastle there are dedicated Sexual Assault Referral Centres where victims can be seen away from A&E and police stations by Sexual Offences Examiners.

History
- Alleged assault and what has happened since
- Basic medical, surgical, and psychiatric history
- Medication—prescribed, over-the-counter, social, drugs of abuse
- Gynaecological, obstetric, and sexual history.

Examination
- Demeanour, intoxication
- Height/weight/BP/pulse/temperature
- General findings
- Injuries (record accurately with diagrams)
  - none
  - bruising
  - abrasions
  - lacerations
  - incisions
  - defence injuries (suggest if typical of specific injuries but avoid conjecture)
- It is important to document both positive and negative findings
- Consider neurological examination
- Auscultation of chest
- Genital, anal, oral, nails
- Keep any other items such as tampons/sanitary towels/condoms in specimen bags if possible or uncontaminated container. Clothes may also be important for evidence.
- Mental state—it is crucially important to assess mental state and risk of suicide or self-harm when assessing anyone presenting with sexual abuse/assault. Conversely victims of abuse frequently present to A&E or psychiatric services with overdoses or deliberate self harm. Previous psychiatric history may determine those at higher risk. Referral to the on-call psychiatric services may be necessary if the victim is judged to be at serious risk of self harm or suicide.

Forensic examination of victims of alleged assaults > 7 days ago for women and > 72 hr for < 13-year-olds and men is unlikely to provide useful evidence and is therefore considered non-urgent. In these circumstances, the health needs should be addressed then they should be referred on to the appropriate services. In most situations this is likely to be the local genitourinary department.

Investigations
Consideration of further investigation by CT or MRI scan, X-ray, or ultrasound may be necessary depending on suspected injuries.

Further management
Any significant bleeding, poisoning or other injuries must be dealt with by usual guidelines and expert help sought. Emergency surgery is occasionally required for genital bleeding or other trauma.

- Emergency contraception[3]: this should be considered and given if there has been any vaginal contact in women or menstruating girls irrespective of stage of menstrual cycle. Current recommendations are for
  - Levonelle 750 µg ×2 stat (to be repeated if vomiting within 3 hours) within 72 hours of sexual act.
  - IUD insertion with antibiotic cover within 5 days (with consideration of cycle and previous intercourse).
- Sexually transmitted infections (STIs)[4]: risk is estimated at 4–56% depending on local prevalence and degree of trauma. If transmitted they may often be multiple. Consider prophylactic antibiotics particularly if unlikely to attend for follow up.
  - 1g azithromycin
  - 500 mg ciprofloxacin
- HIV risk: risk is dependent on prevalence in population and trauma of assault. Consider depending on history but higher risk factors include:
  - assailant HIV positive or in risk group (anal rape of male victims is frequently by heterosexual men)
  - assault within 72 hours
  - anal rape
  - trauma and bleeding
  - multiple assailants

Post-exposure prophylaxis (PEP) is currently 3 antiretroviral drugs. They should be taken as soon as possible (within 1 hr if possible) and within 72 hr. An HIV test is required at baseline and 6 months. Appropriate follow-up must be arranged because of the toxicity of these drugs. There are no studies of the efficacy of PEP after sexual exposure.

The risk of transmission with a single exposure of (higher if traumatic):

- Receptive vaginal intercourse is 1 in 600–2000
- Receptive anal intercourse 1 in 30–150
- Child sexual abuse: early; late/delayed; historic

Most children do not present acutely and may present because of Social Services or medical concerns regarding chronic physical illness/ failure to thrive/neglect.

  - Diagnostic factors for child sexual abuse:
    —Gonorrhoea (if > 1 year)
    —Syphilis and HIV (if congenital infection excluded)
    —Chlamydia (if > 3 years)
  - Factors suspicious of child sexual abuse are:
    —*Trichomonas vaginalis*
    —warts, herpes

Emergency contraception must be remembered acutely in young pubescent girls.

- Follow up:
  - short term-physical wellbeing
  - sexually transmitted infections
  - counselling
  - support services.

Helpline and support services

Rape Crisis: www.rapecrisis.org.uk (local numbers available from website or directory enquiries)

Victim Support: for victims of all crimes including sexual assault www.victimsupport.org.uk
Tel: 0845 30 30 900

Brook: helpline and online enquiry service for the under-25s. www.brook.org.uk Tel: 020 7284 6040

Survivorsuk: for men who have experienced sexual violence www.survivorsuk.org.uk
Tel: 0845 1221201

Rights of Women www.rightsofwomen.org.uk Tel: 020 7251 6577

Suzy Lamplugh Trust: for issues of personal safety www.suzylamplugh.org.uk Tel: 020 8392 1839

Child and Adolescent Mental Health Services (CAMHS): available locally around the UK.

References

1. Sexual Offences Act 2003, Chapter 42, HMSO, London. www.opsi.gov.uk/acts/acts 2003.
2. Wilken J, Welch J (2003). Management of people who have been raped. *BMJ*, **326**, 458–9.
3. FFPRHC Guidance Emergency Contraception (2003). *J Fam Plann Reprod Health Care*, **29**, 9–15. www.ffprhc.org.uk
4. Robinson AJ, Watkeys JEM, Ridgeway GL (1998). Sexually transmitted organisms in sexually abused children. *Arch Dis Child*, **79**, 356–8.

⑦ Pharmacotherapeutics in gynaecology

In gynaecology patients can present as an emergency with the following problems: pelvic inflammatory disease (PID), severe herpes genitalia, menorrhagia, bleeding fibroid, post menopausal bleeding, ectopic pregnancy, miscarriage, torsion of an ovarian cyst, and postoperative complications. The drugs commonly used in these conditions are discussed in the following sections.

Drugs used in the treatment of PID

PID is commonly caused by sexually transmitted infections e.g. *Chlamydia trachomatis*, *Neisseria gonorrhoeae*. It can also be caused by anaerobic organisms and mycoplasma genitalium. It can lead to sub-fertility, ectopic pregnancy, and chronic pelvic pain. Therefore, it should be aggressively treated by multiple drugs. The Royal College of Obstetricians and Gynaecologists recommends the following drug combinations: ofloxacin and metronidazole; cephalosporin, metronidazole and doxycyclin or clindamycin and gentamicin.

Cephalosporins (cefuroxime, cephradine)
- Pharmacology

This group of antibiotics act against the bacteria by inhibiting cell wall synthesis. The mechanism is same as penicillin. There are 4 generations of cephalosporins. Classification by generations is based on general features of antimicrobial activity. Cefuroxime and cephradine belong to the second generation. They are active against Gram-positive as well as Gram-negative organisms.
- Dosage

Cefuroxime:
  - oral 250–500 mg bd
  - IM or IV or infusion—750 mg 6–8 hr, 1.5 mg 6–8 hr in severe infection
  - In surgical prophylaxis 1.5 mg IV at induction.
- Pharmacokinetics

They are excreted primarily by the kidney. Some cephalosporins like cefuroxime can penetrate into CSF. They also cross the placenta.
- Side effects
  - hypersensitivity (about 10% of patients who are allergic to penicillin show cross-reactivity)
  - disturbances in liver enzymes, transient hepatitis and cholestatic jaundice
  - nephrotoxicity.
- Drug interaction
  - probenecid reduces excretion
  - loop diuretics may increase nephrotoxicity.
- Contraindication
  - Hypersensitivity

Doxycycline

● Pharmacology

It is a tetracycline group of drug, which prevent bacterial protein synthesis. They are active against a wide range of Gram-positive and Gram-negative organisms and also chlamydia, mycoplasma, some atypical mytcobacteria.

● Dosage

In PID 100 mg bd for 14 days.

● Pharmacokinetics

Absorption from the gut is 95% (unlike other tetracyclines). Half life is 16–18 hr. It is the only tetracycline which is not excreted in the urine but in the faeces as an inactive conjugate. Hence can be given in renal compromise and there is not much alteration in the intestinal micro flora as well.

● Side effects
  • nausea, vomiting
  • hypersensitivity reaction
  • exacerbation of SLE
  • headache and visual disturbances may indicate benign intracranial hypertension
  • hepatotoxicity.

● Drug interaction
  • antiepileptics increase metabolism of doxycycline
  • doxycycline increases the plasma ciclosporin concentration.

● Contraindication
  • pregnancy, breast-feeding
  • cautious use in alcohol dependence and porphyria.

Macrolides

Erythromycin and azithromycin are the 2 drugs of this group commonly used in gynaecology.

Erythromycin

Is commonly used to treat chlamydial infection in pregnant subjects.

● Pharmacology

This is mainly a bacteriostatic drug, which can be bacteriocidal in high concentration. It acts by inhibiting protein synthesis. It is active against chlamydia and mycoplasma.

● Dosage
  • Oral 250–500 mg every 6 hr
  • IV infusion—50 mg/kg daily by continuous infusion or divided doses every 6 hr.

● Pharmacokinetics

It is incompletely but adequately absorbed from the GI tract. Usually is administered as an enteric-coated tablet as gastric acids inactivate it. It crosses placental barrier. Only 2–5% is excreted by urine, rest is concentrated in liver and excreted in bile.

● Side effects
  • nausea, vomiting, diarrhoea, abdominal discomfort
  • cholestasic jaundice
  • eosinophilia, rashes, urticaria.

- Drug interaction
  - inhibits metabolism of carbamazepine, valproate, midazolam, theophyllin, and methylprednisolone.
  - avoid concomitant use with ergotamine due to risk of ergotism.
  - effect of warfarin is increased.
- Contraindication
Liver disease

Azithromycin

This is another macrolide commonly used because of better patient compliance. In uncomplicated chlamydial infection and nongonococcal urethritis this drug can be used as a single dose (1 g) therapy. This drug is contraindicated in liver diseases.

Clindamycin
- Pharmacology
Suppresses protein synthesis. Usually used in cases of penicillin sensitivity.
- Dosage
  - oral: 150–300 mg 6 hrly
  - deep IM or IV infusion 0.6–2.7 g daily in 2–4 divided doses. May be increased to 4.8 g daily in life-threatening infections. Single IV dose not to exceed 1.2 g.
- Pharmacokinetics
Almost completely absorbed from the gut. Half-life 2.9 hr. It easily crosses placenta. Excreted in urine and bile.
- Side effects
Serious toxic effect is antibiotic associated colitis.
- Drug interaction
  - increases the effect of non-depolarizing muscle relaxants.
  - antagonises the effect of neogstigmine and pyridostigmine.
- Contraindication
Diarrhoeal state

Aminoglycosides

These are a group of bactericidal drugs, which act by interfering with the protein synthesis. They are mainly active against aerobic Gram-negative bacteria. Though they are widely used, serious toxicity is a major limitation to their usefulness. During therapy drug concentration in blood has to be monitored. Gentamicin, amikacin, neomycin, natilmicin, streptomycin, and tobramycin belong to this group.

Gentamicin

It is one of the most commonly used aminoglycosides.
- Use
Septicaemia, meningitis, and other CNS infections, acute pyelonephritis, biliary infection, pneumonia, endocarditis. It has a broad spectrum but is inactive against anaerobes and has poor activity against haemolytic streptococci and pneumococci. When used for 'blind' treatment in undiagnosed serious infection, it is used with penicillin or metronidazole or both.

- Dosage

3–5 mg/kg in divided doses, usually 8 hrly. Loading and maintenance doses are calculated on the basis of patient's weight and renal function and are adjusted according to serum concentration of gentamicin.

- Pharmacokinetics

They are very poorly absorbed from the GI tract, but rapidly absorbed from the IM sites of injection. Excretion is almost exclusively by glomerular IM filtration, half-life being 2–3 hr.

- Side effects
  - nephrotoxicity
  - ototoxicity
  - hypomagnesaemia on prolonged therapy.
- Drug interaction
  - indomethacin increases plasma concentration
  - increased risk of nephrotoxicity with amphotericin, ciclosporin, cisplatin
  - increased ototoxicity with loop diuretics.
- Contraindication

Myasthenia gravis

Quinolones (ciprofloxacin, ofloxacin)

They are bactericidal agents, which act by interfering with bacterial DNA synthesis.

- Dosage
  - ciprofloxacin: oral: 500–750 mg bd
    Uncomplicated gonorrhoea 500 mg single dose
    IV 200–400 mg bd (400 mg over 60 min)
  - Ofloxacin: oral: uncomplicated gonorrhoea 400 mg single dose
    PID 400 mg bd for 14 days
    IV 400 mg bd (400 mg over 60 min)
- Pharmacokinetics

Well-absorbed after oral administration. Ofloxacin and ciprofloxacin are eliminated by kidney.

- Side effects
  - nausea vomiting, abdominal pain, diarrhoea
  - rashes, pruritus
  - headache, dizziness
  - rare but serious hepatic damage can occur
  - renal failure, nephritis
  - ofloxacin can cause hypotension, neuropathy, extrapyramidal symptoms etc.
- Drug interaction
  - increased risk of convulsions with NSAID and theophyllins
  - opioid analgesics reduce plasma concentration of ciprofloxacin
  - antacids, sucralfate, calcium and irons reduce absorption
  - quinolones increase anticoagulant effects of warfarin and acenocoumarol
  - plasma concentration of phenytoin is altered.
- Contraindications

Cautious use in conditions predisposing to seizures, renal impairment, myasthenia.

Metronidazole
- Pharmacology

It is a nitroimidazole group of drug. Usually used in PID. It is also commonly used in suspected anaerobic infections and for prophylaxis in surgery.
- Dosage
  - oral 400 mg tds
  - IV 500 mg 8 hrly.
- Pharmacokinetics

Mainly metabolized in the liver and excreted in urine. Half-life is 8 hr.
- Side effects
  - nausea, vomiting, unpleasant taste
  - rashes
  - abnormal LFTs
  - urticaria and erythema multiforme in cases of hypersensitivity
  - peripheral neuropathy in cases of prolonged use.
- Drug interactions

Alcohol—disulfirum like reaction.

Genital herpes
Acyclovir

- Pharmacology

It is an antiviral drug active mainly against herpes virus. It acts by inhibiting viral DNA synthesis. This drug is effective only if started at the onset of the disease.
- Use

Generally used in genital herpes and chicken pox/shingles.
- Dosage
  - 200 mg 5 times a day for 5 days.
  - 800 mg 5 times a day is used in cases of varicella and herpes zoster.
  - IV infusion is used in immunocompromised, severe initial genital herpes and varicella zoster. 5 mg/kg bodyweight every 8 hr for 5 days.
- Pharmacokinetics

Oral bioavailability is 10%–30%. Renal excretion is the principal source of elimination.
- Side effect
  - GI disturbances, hepatitis, jaundice
  - headache, neurological reactions
  - hypersensitivity reaction
  - acute renal failure.
- Drug interaction
  - probenecid reduces excretion
  - higher concentration with concomitant administration.

Menorrhagia and dysmenorrhoea
Antifibrinolytic drug

Tranexamic acid

Tranexamic acid is a fibrinolytic agent, which prevents bleeding by inhibiting fibrinolysis. It is one of the commonest used drugs in cases of menorrhagia.

- Dosage

1g 3–4 times daily in menorrhagia when heavy bleeding has started.
- Side effects
  - nausea, vomiting, diarrhoea
  - disturbances in colour vision (to stop the drug)
  - thromboembolic events
- Contraindications

Thromboembolic disease

NSAIDs

The commonly used analgesics in gynaecology are NSAIDs. They have the advantage of being effective in cases of dysmenorrhoea and menorrhagia. The opioid analgesics are used mainly in the postoperative period.

Mefenamic acid

- Pharmacology

It is an NSAID with minimal anti-inflammatory effect. It is mainly used in dysmenorrhoea with menorrhagia.
- Dosage

500 mg tds preferably after food.
- Pharmacokinetics
  - plasma half-life is 2–4 hr
  - 50% is excreted in urine.
- Side effects
  - GI problems are the commonest ones—dyspepsia or discomfort
  - diarrhoea (may need discontinuation of treatment)
  - thrombocytopenia, haemolytic anaemia (positive Coombs' test) and aplastic anaemia
  - convulsion with overdose.
- Drug interaction
  - avoid concomitant use of 2 NSAIDs
  - anticoagulant effect of warfarin is enhanced
  - excretion of lithium is reduced.
- Contraindications
  - inflammatory bowel disease
  - hypersensitivity to aspirin and NSAIDs
  - peptic ulcer.

Diclofenac

Used mainly as an analgesic

- Pharmacology

It is an anti-inflammatory, antipyretic, and analgesic agent. It is an inhibitor of cyclooxygenase.
- Dosage
  - orally 75–150 mg in 2–3 divided doses, preferably after food.
  - deep IM injection into the gluteal muscle, 75 mg od for maximum 2 days.
  - rectal suppositories—75–150 mg daily in divided doses.

- Pharmacokinetics

Rapidly and completely absorbed after oral administration. There is substantial first pass effect and only 50% of diclofenac is available systemically. Plasma half-life is 1–2 hr. Metabolites are excreted in urine (65%) and bile (35%).

- Side effects
  - GI discomfort, nausea, diarrhoea, bleeding, ulceration
  - hypersensitivity reaction
  - headache, dizziness, drowsiness
  - blood disorders, renal failure, especially in pre-existing renal impairment
  - hepatic damage.
- Drug interactions

Excretion of methotrexate reduced by diclofenac causing toxicity (see Mefenamic acid).

- Contraindications
  - porphyria
  - hypersensitivity
  - active peptic ulcer.

Hormonal preparations

A variety of hormonal preparations are used in gynaecology to treat heavy periods. Some of them are used to control acute loss.

GnRh analogues (goserelin, leuprorelin)

- Pharmacology

Luteinizing hormone, follicle stimulating hormone, and chorionic gonadotrophin are glycoprotein family of hormones referred to as gonadotrophin hormones as they act on the gonads. Pituitary gonadotrophin secretion is stimulated by gonadotrophin releasing hormone (GnRh). A number of clinically useful GnRh analogues have been synthesized.

- Use

They are used in endometriosis, infertility and most importantly in controlling severely bleeding fibroid.

- Dosage
  - goserelin—3.6 mgs monthly
  - leuprorelin 3.75 mg sc or im monthly.
- Side effects
  - menopausal symptoms
  - decrease in trabecular bone density if used for more than 6 months
  - headache
  - hypersensitivity reaction
  - fibroid degeneration can occur.
- Contraindications
  - should not be used for > 6 months
  - undiagnosed vaginal bleeding
  - pregnancy and breast-feeding.

GnRh antagonist (cetrorelix)
- this new drug is a luteinising hormone releasing hormone (LHRH) antagonist. It competitively blocks the binding of LHRH to pituitary gonadotrophin releasing hormone receptors, resulting in suppression of secretion of gonadotrophins.
- used in treatment of endometriosis and ovarian stimulation in cases of fertility treatment.
- usually administered by SC route.
- occasionally can present with skin reactions.

Oestrogen
Oestrogen preparations are not used in emergency gynaecology. Previously they were used in treating acute menorrhagia (puberty menorrhagia). However, it is no longer used because of the risk of venous thrombosis. Oestrogen alone is only used in HRT after hysterectomy.

Progestogens
Progestogens were widely used in menorrhagia but they are not effective in reducing heavy loss. They are effective in irregular bleeding when taken cyclically from D5 to D26 of the cycle. Nowadays they are mainly used for HRT, contraception, and in cancers and hence have limited use in emergency gynaecology.

Medical treatment of ectopic pregnancy

Methotrexate is used in medical management of ectopic pregnancy.

Methotrexate
- Pharmacology
It is an antimetabolite and acts by inhibiting the enzyme dihydrofolate reductase which is essential in purine and pyrimidine synthesis.
- Use
It can be used in ectopic pregnancy in the following conditions
  - β HCG level is < 3000 U/L
  - there is no cardiac activity in the ectopic pregnancy
  - minimal symptoms
  - regular follow-ups can be ensured (risk of rupture in 7%).
About 15% of patients may need repeat dosage.
- Dosage
Most commonly used dosage is a single dose of 50 mg/m.
- Pharmacokinetics
It is rapidly absorbed from the GI tract at smaller dosage (< 25 mg/m^2), but larger doses are not well-absorbed, and should be administered intravenously. About 90% of the drug is excreted unchanged in urine.
- Side effects
  - myelosuppression
  - mucositis
  - rarely pneumonitis
  - (Folinic acid following methotrexate helps to prevent mucositis or myelosuppression).

- Drug interactions
  - increased toxicity with aspirin and NSAIDs, ciclosporin, corticosteroid, acitretin.
  - anti-folate effect enhanced by cotrimoxazole and trimethoprim, phenytoin, pyrimethamine.
  - excretion reduced by penicillins, sulphonamides, probenecid.
- Contraindications
  - significant renal and hepatic impairment
  - presence of fetal cardiac activity within the ectopic mass
  - active infection
  - immunodeficiency syndrome
  - pregnancy (to avoid conception for 6 months after stopping)
  - caution in porphyria.

Further Reading

1. Goodman and Gilman's The Pharmacological Basis of Therapeutics by Hardman J.G., Limbire L.E and Gilman A.G. 10th Edition Mc Graw Hill August 2001
2. British National Formulary September 2005, Published by British Medical Association. BMJ Publishing Group Ltd. Tavistock Square, London.
3. Management of Acute Pelvic Inflammatory Disease, May 2003. (Clinical Green Top Guideline No 32) Published by Royal College of Obstetricians and Gynaecologists.

Index